Clinical Supervision

2nd edition

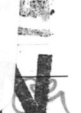

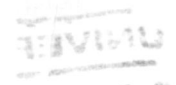

ESSENTIALS OF NURSING MANAGEMENT

Series Editor: Jill Baker

The complexity and changing status of the National Health Service demands that all key professional staff are accountable for both their practice and for the efficient and effective deployment of human and physical resources. The series equips nurses and midwives with the knowledge and skills essential for the application of effective managerial and leadership practice. The series focuses on a range of significant management issues that confront and challenge practising nurses, managers and educationalists working within both hospital and primary care settings.

All books in the series:

Essentials of Nursing Management
Series Standing Order:
ISBN: 1–4039–4597–7
(outside North America only)

You can receive future titles in this series as they are published, by placing a standing order. Please contact your bookseller, or, in the case of difficulty, write to us at the address below with your name and address, the title of the series, and the ISBN quoted above.

Customer Services Department, Palgrave Ltd, Houndmills, Basingstoke, Hampshire, RG21 6XS, England

CLINICAL SUPERVISION IN PRACTICE

Some Questions, Answers and Guidelines for Professionals in Health and Social Care

2ND EDITION

Edited by

Veronica Bishop

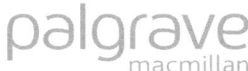

First edition 1997
Reprinted: 1998, 2000, 2006
Second edition 2007 published by
PALGRAVE MACMILLAN
Houndmills, Basingstoke, Hampshire RG21 6XS and
175 Fifth Avenue, New York, N.Y. 10010
Companies and representatives throughout the world.

PALGRAVE MACMILLAN is the global academic imprint of the Palgrave
Macmillan division of St. Martin's Press, LLC and of Palgrave Macmillan Ltd.
Macmillan® is a registered trademark in the United States, United Kingdom
and other countries. Palgrave is a registered trademark in the European
Union and other countries.

ISBN-13: 978–1–4039–9301–4
ISBN-10: 1–4039–9301–7

This book is printed on paper suitable for recycling and made from fully
managed and sustained forest sources.

A catalogue record for this book is available from the British Library.

10   9   8   7   6   5   4   3   2   1
16 15 14 13 12 11 10 09 08 07

Printed and bound in China

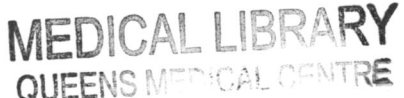

Contents

List of Figures, Tables and Boxes

List of Figures

Tables

Boxes

Foreword

I have been involved in nursing for more years than I wish to remember, as a nurse, district nurse, manager, regional nurse and now as the Chief Nursing Officer for England. One of the pitfalls of growing older is looking back at the past through rose tinted spectacles, recalling the golden years of nursing when caring and dedication were all that mattered and patients were better cared for – and did as they were told!

Every day I meet nurses and patients in many different care settings and I often think about the long way that our profession has come. I am struck by the breadth and depth and diversity of the work and the myriad of opportunities open to nurses today. Increasingly the nurse is the pivotal person in a patient's care – a familiar and tested role in a world of new and confusing titles.

One of the successes in recent years is that we are better at explaining what nursing is all about and getting the core values of nursing embedded in the heart of the NHS. Today we hear care, dignity, respect, privacy, safety, and cleanliness spoken by politicians, doctors, chief executives, nurse leaders and the public. I believe that this change has been driven as much by the public as by the profession. Patients know what good care means and they know how important it is, they also know when it isn't right.

In many ways health care is becoming more complicated. Public expectations are changing. Patients want a greater role in their own care and for services to meet their individual needs. Nursing work is more demanding as the number of people with acute and multiple conditions, both physical and mental, increase and society gets older. In this complex world it is more important than ever that nurses are supported in their everyday practice. Nurses need space and opportunity to understand the process of care and to think about the, often messy, world of the nurse/patient relationship. Knowing oneself is the first step in being able to care for others and clinical supervision is a key tool in that journey.

I have seen new models, titles and concepts come and go in nursing over the years. Nonetheless, clinical supervision remains an enduring part of good nursing practice because of its central role in safeguarding patients, improving care and empowering nurses. In this book Veronica Bishop peels back the layers to uncover the core of what clinical supervision means and gives us useful examples of how it works in practice. I am sure this book, now in its second edition, will do much to keep clinical supervision on the agenda of busy, dedicated nurses and their organisations.

Prof. Chris Beasley, Chief Nursing Officer

Preface

What is in my view, incontrovertible, is the potential power of nurses, and what amazes me is their reluctance to take hold of it.

While it is a great pleasure to build on the first edition of this book, drawing in and building on the substantial body of work that has been carried out in the intervening 8 years, it is none the less a sad reflection of the times that for many clinical supervision is still merely a name, a philosophy that never made it past the headlines. Despite the paucity of good clinical supervision implementation programmes there has been a growing number of books, papers and articles on clinical supervision over the past 12 years or so, much stemming from the United Kingdom but with some significant work from Australia, the United States and Scandinavia. The significance of these works is the overarching recognition that some mechanism is missing from the philosophical framework of nursing to support the provision of excellence in care. Experience of facilitating the introduction of clinical supervision to a wide range of clinical areas and differing levels of seniority over many years has shown me that many well-meaning attempts to introduce supervision tend to 'peter out' over time, except where there is strong managerial commitment to it. Cottrell and Smith (2003) also found this and looked to the field of interpersonal dynamics for an explanation, describing a relationship rhombus to provide a framework of understanding and discussion. Not surprisingly, they identified that issues such as constant change, tensions between different levels of management as well as inadequate preparation for clinical supervision all contrive to prevent its effective implementation. This somewhat flies in the face of the work by Perron et al. (2005) who have suggested that nursing as a profession is at the heart of bio power in that nurses lie at the cross roads between the biological and political ranges of power over life. These authors postulate that nurses are at the flexing point between state requirements and those of the individual, thus occupying a strategic position to act as instruments of government. If this is the case, can one equally argue the case for nurses being in a position to be instrumental contrary to state ideologies? What is, in my view, incontrovertible is the potential power of nurses, and what amazes me is their reluctance to take hold of it. This must stem from unclear leadership, and unshared values and strategies to achieve those values. I have stated elsewhere (Bishop, 2004) that in recent years no one has consolidated the attention of the nursing profession and maintained that attention. By the same token, few leaders have fully embraced clinical supervision, as the game of catch up with government is too absorbing, and meantime practitioners are badly neglected.

So does this matter? If individuals can carve out careers for themselves that satisfy them, if quality control is handed to various agencies, and if nursing as a profession disappears into the integrated woodwork while generic health care workers pick up the hands on aspects of health care, perhaps nursing as it has been identified over the last century is no longer needed. There has been a strong move from various governments over the past 20 years to reduce professional dominance in health care, with considerable success. This success has been particularly notable with nurses who have been lured with sweet words of team work and integrated working, as well as higher salaries, away from a rather patriarchal medical dominance into a management hierarchy. Sadly, these structures often have little connection with patients and more in common with Sainsbury's! Many fine nurses suffered badly as a result of this swift courtship, being cast off from the team as soon as the next tranche of organisational changes came along. Patriarchy from our medical colleagues possibly had a little more going for it! For good or otherwise the general move of health care staff into teams, combined with ever changing needs of the public in response to new developments and treatments, has blurred disciplinary boundaries. Chronic shortages of registered nurses, the majority of whom are female and many of whom are bringing up young families or caring for elderly relatives are compounded by an aging population. Perhaps then it is not surprising that a major European study currently ongoing, with data from over half a million nurses indicates that the United Kingdom has the highest percentage of nurses who regularly consider leaving nursing (Hasselhorn, 2005). Despite this, it must also be said that for some individuals wonderful opportunities have been grasped, and dynamic ways of providing services are evolving, but rarely within an overarching strategy, and sometimes with little collegiate support. These can be exciting times, but as Butterworth observed (1998, p.180) the need to surround these new ways of working with safe, supportive supervision and debate is equally important.

So where do we go from here? The nursing profession is at a very important point in its development and one that requires careful consideration if it is not just to survive but to grow. 'We consider this point of time to be of particular significance, perhaps on a par with the Registration Act of 1919, because wrong footedness in the next few years will see the demise of a noble concept' (Freshwater and Bishop, 2004; p. 196). Nursing lacks the coherence of other care disciplines – its positive strength in being fluid and responsive can too easily become a source of professional destruction. Now we seem to be caught in a web of strong threads that stem from such sources as gender stereotyping, political game playing, resource deprivation and inadequate professional leadership at many levels (Collinson, 2003; Freshwater, 2002; Marriner, 1994), which conspire to keep us in the place where others would have us. Individuals can, and do, cut through some of this, but the real swathe cutting has to be highly visible. Nurses have a poor record of supporting each other, another reason why we have provided an easy target for those seeking to marginalize us. If the arguments offered by Perron et al (2005) have any substance let clinical supervision be the result of the bio power. The contributors to this book are all renowned professionals and bring their own power to the reader. We are all committed to making clinical supervision a reality for every practitioner, and hope that this book will help that to happen. Why? Read on, and you will see!

References

Bishop V, Freshwater D (2004) Looking ahead. In: Freshwater D, Bishop V (eds) *Nursing Research in Context: Appreciation, Application and Personal Development*. Palgrave, Basingstoke. p. 196.

Bishop V (2004) Editorial. *Journal of Research in Nursing* (formerly *Nursing Times Research*), 9(3).

Butterworth T (1998) Clinical supervision; what is it? In: Bishop V (ed.) *Clinical Supervision in Practice: Some Questions, Answers and Guidelines*. Macmillan/NTResearch, Basingstoke.

Collinson G (2003) The primacy of purpose and the leadership of nursing. *NTResearch*, 7(6): 403–411.

Cottrell S and Georgina Smith (2003) www.clinical-supervision/ default.htm

Freshwater D (2002) *Therapeutic Nursing: Improving Patient Care Through Reflection.* Sage, London.

Hasselhorn H et al. (2005) NEXT-Study. University of Wuppertal and Unjiversity of Witten, Germany. www.next.uni-wuppertal.de/ results_eng.htm

Marriner AC (1994) Theories of leadership. In: Hein CF and Nicholson MJ (eds) *Contemporary Leadership Behaviour* (4th ed) Lippincot Co., Philadelphia

Perron A, Fluct C and Holmes D (2005) Agents of care and agents of the state:bio power and nursing practice. *J Adv. Nurs.,* 50(5): 536.

Acknowledgements

Jerome Carson will always be indebted to Professors Butterworth and Bishop for inviting him to contribute to the Clinical Supervision Evaluation Project. He would also like to thank Dr Julie Winstanley for providing him with a copy of the Manchester Scale.

This book is dedicated to the memory of John Newson, and acknowledges with gratitude the unstinting generosity and support of colleagues who share my passion for nursing.

Notes on the Contributors

Veronica Bishop Veronica is Editor in Chief of the Journal of Research in Nursing and Visiting Professor at Bournemouth University. She is also a board member of the Hong Kong nurses' journal; a member of the scientific committee for the RCN Research Society and until recently was an executive member of the Florence Nightingale Foundation and a member of its academic panel. After undertaking clinical research at the Royal College of Surgeons (England) and obtaining an MPhil, followed by a Doctorate from London University she joined the Civil Service as a Nursing Officer in the Department of Health (DH). At the DH she was responsible for a large body of research specifically related to nursing and all health disciplines manpower. She also had the national lead on clinical supervision, commissioning the first national multi-site study in nursing. Veronica has worked as a consultant for the WHO in Denmark, India and Romania, and is widely published and has presented keynote speeches at numerous nursing conferences. She is currently working with the Prison Services on implementing clinical supervision, and continues to support activities in this area.

Dr Jerome Carson is employed as Consultant Clinical Psychologist within the Lambeth Directorate of the South London and Maudsley NHS Trust. He is Honorary Senior Lecturer at King's College London, Institute of Psychiatry. Jerome did his psychology degree at Reading University, his clinical training at the University of East London and his doctorate at King's College. He has written or co-edited four books, most recently *Be Your Own Self-Esteem Coach*, published by Whiting and Birch. He has written over 100 papers or book chapters. His main research interests have been in the field of staff stress and health services research. He was a core member of the Clinical Supervision Evaluation Project, directed by Professor Butterworth, which was one of the largest studies ever conducted into the effects of clinical supervision on staff.

Philip Esterhuizen is Senior Lecturer, IHCS, Bournemouth University. He is the lead researcher and facilitator in the Dorset

Academic Centres in Practice, where he uses confluent teaching and learning approaches to engage practitioners and managers in continuous improvement processes. He is a skilled supervisor and is currently involved in facilitating action-learning sets to develop supervisory training.

Dawn Freshwater is Professor of Mental Health and Director of the Centre for Applied Research in Mental Health and Primary Care, IHCS, Bournemouth University. She is the Editor of the *Journal of Psychiatric Mental Health Nursing* and President of the International Association for Human Caring. As a Fellow of the Royal College of Nursing she has 25 years experience in teaching, practicing and researching in health care settings. Her research has included work related to reflective practice and clinical supervision, which was the subject of her PhD study in 1998.

Liz Henderson is Lead Cancer Nurse for Northern Ireland Cancer Network and Lead Nurse for Cancer Services at Belfast City Hospital Trust. She provides strategic nurse leadership in the development of nursing for people affected by cancer, and in the creation of multi-professional cancer networks. Working in partnership with the network team she helps to develop and co-ordinate implementation of cancer service development plans. In addition she is responsible for nurse leadership at the Regional Cancer Centre based at Belfast City Hospital Trust in the ongoing development of effective person centred cancer services. Liz serves on a number of policy committees and development groups in these areas. She has a particular interest in facilitation as a means of enabling the development of practice, and is interested in ways to maximise learning in the workplace

Brendan McCormack is Professor of Nursing Research, Institute of Nursing Research, University of Ulster. He is also Director of Nursing Research and Practice Development, Royal Hospitals Trust, Belfast; Adjunct Professor of Nursing, Faculty of Medicine, Nursing and Health Care, Monash University, Melbourne, Australia; and Visiting Professor, School of Health, Communication & Education Studies, University of Northumbria, Newcastle, England. He leads the Institute of Nursing Research 'Working with Older People' Recognised Research Group, coordinating research and development activity in this area. His writing and research work focuses on gerontological nursing and practice development and he serves on a number of editorial boards, policy committees, and development groups in these areas. He has a particular focus on the use of arts and creativity in healthcare research and development. He is the co-editor of the *International Journal of Older People Nursing*.

Elizabeth Walsh is a researcher practitioner in prison health care, IHCS, Bournemouth University. She has facilitated and researched the implementation of clinical supervision and reflective practice across the prison health care setting and is currently undertaking her PhD using reflexive methodologies that incorporate clinical supervision as a data collection tool.

1

Clinical Supervision: What Is It? Why Do We Need It?

Veronica Bishop

SYNOPSIS

This chapter sets out the professional and policy reasons for the inclusion of clinical supervision on the national nursing agenda. The impact that clinical supervision offers the individual practitioner in supporting professional aims, and its role in meeting high standards of care is highlighted. What clinical supervision is, and what it is *not* is discussed and working definitions are given. The text highlights that clinical supervision is about empowerment of the individual, and stresses the need for professional development. The importance of clinical supervision within the context of clinical governance is explained, and the ethical tensions are discussed.

Introduction

> Clinical supervision – is a designated interaction between two or more practitioners within a safe and supportive environment, that enables a continuum of reflective critical analysis of care, to ensure quality patients services, and the well being of the practitioner.
>
> (Bishop and Sweeney, 2006)

How do nurses and other health care professionals know that they are practising in a safe, effective and professionally enriching way? And how or where do they get the professional support to develop their role when they need it? 'How do you know what you don't know?' Clinical supervision has been suggested as the answer to many of the challenges facing nursing today and in the foreseeable future, but how many, rather than just having heard the term, really understand

what it could mean to them? In this chapter, I will unpick the begin-
nings, the middle and the ongoing conversation about clinical supervision, over ten years old now, but still alive and kicking hard, and
illustrate where the individual nurse and the profession as a whole
can take it to their benefit. Make no mistake, the individual can make
their mark here, if they are sufficiently moved – and I do hope that
they will be! My entire aim for this book is to get practitioners to say
'give it to me' ' I will not work without it' 'I am worth this!'

There must be times in all our working lives when we read the
latest edict from the centre, or from our professional colleagues
expressing yet another concept, and think – oh yes, another quick
fix, another piece of jargon! Let me cite an example. In my 30 years
plus of nursing the notion of the 'nursing process', 'individualized
patient care', 'holistic care planning', 'seamless care', 'named nurse' –
to name but a few – have been labels for person-centred care and
hailed as the ideal way forward. And yet it seems that care is far
from individualised, and patients are often very unhappy at the
hands of what in some instances has become a very depersonalized
health care system. So why should you, the reader, spend precious
time digesting yet another concept – what can clinical supervision
do for you? If you care enough for yourself and your work it can
change your professional life, giving you the confidence to relate
therapeutically and with empathy to patients, and make those
patients feel that they are known to you. You will have the resources
within yourself to comfort and care for the patient who thinks:

> It will be dark one night, and someone's nurses will be tiptoeing
> outside my room. I will be lying there, in the bed that you made
> for me; I will be scared and wondering if I am safe – will I die here?
> Do you know I am here? Do you know my name? (Berwick, 2004)

Berwick acknowledged the tremendous power of nursing, set
against the fragility of the relationship with an individual patient.
For nursing to realise that power, and to use it in a therapeutic way
is surely what being a professional provider of health care is about.
But how to achieve this? What framework will consistently support
each individual nurse or healthcare worker in balancing their workload, in feeling empathy with their patients and clients despite a fast
turnover, and in driving forward standards of care without burning
out? I believe that properly implemented, clinical supervision can
help us to achieve this.

Do I put too much into the value of clinical supervision? Professor Tony Butterworth, with whom I have worked on promoting clinical supervision for over a decade, once laughingly informed a conference at which we were both presenting, that I had never had clinical supervision! It is precisely for that reason that I strive to make sure that others do have the benefit of it. I hope that they are never in the position I was in when, to take one example, on an intensive care course in a major London hospital, I admitted a child so badly sexually abused that she died, and when I was found in tears after all the clinical processes had been carried out, I was quickly sent home for a half day – in case I upset the other nurses! Or the time when, new to the intensive therapeutic unit (ITU), I successfully resuscitated a man who had suffered cardiac arrest, to be told that I had been overenthusiastic – he was not for resuscitation! The pain and frustration of such instances are not unique to me, we have probably all been in similar situations in our time, but that doesn't mean that there is nothing to be learned from them. How important is it to anyone dealing with people in often fraught circumstances to mirror what they are doing, to 'play back' and reflect on current practices, to self-critique and to grow both personally and professionally? Very important – indeed crucial for any thinking practitioner – and this reflection is most effective if done with peers, a person, or people who have some understanding of what you need to achieve and how to succeed in those goals.

Nursing is not the only area of work where some form of feedback, self-help or simple support is considered beneficial. Buddy systems and mentorship arrangements, for example, are not uncommon in many industrial organisations, and are becoming more and more accepted as the norm. What perhaps is a little more specific in clinical supervision is the element of peer review and supportive challenge which, in good partnerships, brings out the sharpness in clinical practice – that extra awareness which derives from shared learning with colleagues. However, what must be kept clearly in the mind of the reader is that registered nurses or midwives are personally accountable for their practice (UKCC, 1992) and that while clinical supervision offers a framework to support the practitioner in their professional accountability, it does not shift that accountability to another.

An important starting place for the newcomer to the subject of clinical supervision is an understanding of what is meant by it, and why it is on the nursing agenda. Perversely perhaps, I think that a definition will be more useful to the reader *after* the reasons for its introduction are explained. This chapter will provide the recent history and current rationale for implementing clinical supervision, and will then go on to discuss many of the published definitions, unpicking some of the misconceptions that surround the topic.

Policy and Professional Drivers

There were many reasons why, in the 1990s, clinical supervision ceased to be an activity barely heard of and only practised in elite corners of the nursing profession, such as in mental health, where nurses had adapted the concept from their experiences of psychotherapy. These reasons are worth recalling, as their nature, those being organisational instability, fast turnover of patients and increased workload have not changed, nor are they likely to.

The most obvious and dramatic change in nursing was the reorganisation of its education with the introduction of Project 2000 (UKCC, 1986). This initiative paved the way to move nurse education from schools of nursing, generally attached to hospitals, to institutions of higher education. The very work specific but academically fairly worthless Registered General Nurse (RGN) was reconfigured to fit a more academically able nurse who had achieved diploma or degree status. The old apprenticeship model of learning was fading, not only because it did not fit with the current ethos of a thinking and questioning practitioner, rather than a process-orientated one, but because staff shortages and fast turnover of patients meant there were fewer opportunities for newly qualified staff to observe experienced staff at work. This 'being thrown in at the deep end' approach to workforce management resulted in a high staff turnover rate in nursing, and poor overall retention, a situation already well documented (Buchan, 2003, 2004). It was also, and still is, counterproductive to supporting staff in decision-making, innovation and autonomy of practice, the supposed by-products of higher education. Woods (1992, p. 41) summed this up neatly when he stated:

> This climate of increased managerialism and cash limiting of services imposes tremendous stresses on nurses attempting to have an open and helpful relationship with their patients. The danger is that many aspects of nursing care are simply impossible to carry

out. Constraints on time and external pressures impose impossible demands. In busy acute wards it is quite common for nurses to return from their two days off and not know any of the patients on their ward. The question must seriously be asked, what is this doing to the ability of the nurse to care appropriately and adequately for the patient?

Not only was nursing changing to meet new technologies and new demands, the NHS was undergoing yet another major change, with the introduction of an internal market system. This purchaser–provider split was seen by the Conservative Thatcher government of the day as a way of ensuring that funding in the NHS followed the patient and would separate the running of hospitals from their financing. Other proposals in the White Paper Working for Patients (1989) accelerated changes in management, and the universal application of audit mechanisms. It was also the introduction to issues around reducing junior doctors' hours that were to have a major impact on nursing. [Readers with an interest in a more in-depth study of these changes will enjoy Webster's excellent book on the history of the NHS (2002).]

In 1994, a Department of Health (DoH) commissioned Position Paper on clinical supervision by Faugier and Butterworth (1994) was circulated widely in the NHS and the independent sector, with an accompanying letter by the then Chief Nursing Officer for England. This stated that she considered clinical supervision to be fundamental to safeguarding standards and to the development of professional expertise for the delivery of quality care (DoH, 1994). The Position Paper was also distributed in Scotland and the two countries were to liaise closely in achieving some consensus on the way forward in the implementation of clinical supervision (Davidson, 1998). Wales also took the concept forward, as did Northern Ireland. Further central support for the initiative was indicated in the government's review on mental health nursing (DoH, 1994) circulated a year later. The fact that clinical supervision became a UK-wide initiative reflected the need felt by the profession as a whole that something was needed to support practitioners through the many changes which were being thrust upon them – and indeed still are and are likely to continue to be – while they endeavour to provide the best care possible. As the lead DoH nursing officer at that time for clinical supervision I led multiple centrally funded workshops and conferences across the country to engage with the profession on

the concept of clinical supervision, its principles and potential benefits. Trust nurse executives contributed greatly to the debate and
reached a consensus that clinical supervision is about empowering
the practitioner, and that management should support it as it offers
a framework for public safely and clinical excellence (Butterworth
and Bishop, 1994). However, despite the involvement of Trust nurse
executives it is cogently argued (Grant and Townend; in press) that
the tensions between macro and micro organisational and cultural
factors have not been properly addressed. These both simultaneously can give rise to the need for clinical supervision and undermine its uptake. The authors argue that those wishing to champion
clinical supervision would do well to increase their awareness of
these issues, a view that I fully support.

Despite this apparent commitment, Driscoll (2000) noted that
implementation has been a struggle, not least because many practitioners are unclear as to what it is. Power (1999) wrote that as a practitioner desperately seeking clinical supervision he was initially
regarded by his colleagues as something of an oddity – until his
improved practice became noticeable. He also commented that a
major problem during his early supervision experiences was that no
one ever told him how to be supervised. This book will address that
major issue in Chapter 4. Power was not alone in his difficulty, and
it is likely that lack of practical information on how to implement
clinical supervision has been one of the main reasons why practitioners did not push to take part in it, and why managers have not
pushed to resource it. Hindsight is a wonderful thing! Many nurses
at both management and practitioner level have said that it would
have helped in the implementation if the centre (DoH) had been
more prescriptive. That this may have had major resource implications for the government may have been one reason for the reti-
cence, another was the genuine desire from both the DoH and the
United Kingdom Central Council (UKCC) for the profession to
develop clinical supervision as it saw fit. A further block to the
implementation of clinical supervision is the self-fulfilling but self-
defeating prophecy of 'I can't change anything', 'what difference
will it make?' Pearson (1998) noted that as a profession we have continual difficulty in moving forward, stemming from our tendency to
polarize. Bond and Holland (1998) acknowledged such cynicism
and the 'so what's new?' attitude that many have towards clinical
supervision but rightly challenge it. They considered that we are all
destined to keep on repeating ourselves, both individually and

collectively as a profession, until what is being aimed for is understood and attainable, stating:

> This cannot happen until the powerful processes which inhibit us from understanding and reaching perceived ... goals are also acknowledged, accepted and understood. In doing so we divest them of their power to sabotage the process. (p. 43)

They discussed what they term the hidden picture – resistance to clinical supervision which may relate to fears of power and autonomy, and fear of developing professional relationships, not generally part of the anti-emotional climate of the nursing profession, a view touched on by Faugier (1992). Fowler (1996) argued that nursing as a profession must and is developing its own body of theory on which nurses make choices about practice and are responsible for the outcomes of their actions. He muted that while this can be taught in the classroom practice can only be mastered through supervised practice. This stance could argue for a didactic approach (I suspect not his intention) with overt supervision in practice, which differs from the theoretical stance taken by Johns, who promoted a process of guided reflection (Johns, 1998). Despite the lack of nationwide clarity, the cynicism and the resistance to professional development offered through clinical supervision, the concept has been, and is still promoted from our more visionary and possibly more stubborn colleagues. They have identified it as, at worst, a mechanism to safeguard minimum clinical standards and public safety, and at best to sustain and develop excellence in practice. I have previously warned colleagues that

> while clinical supervision will help nurses to achieve the best level of care possible, it cannot compensate for inadequate facilities, poor management or unmotivated staff. However it will create a culture within which nurses can flourish if they are willing to embrace it, and if management is supportive. (Bishop, 1994; p. 36)

Over a decade later I strongly suggest that stubborn commitment is essential to overcome the barriers to implementing clinical supervision. For while the combination of staff shortages, overburdened staff and lack of funds and or facilities provide compelling reasons to give up on it, they are, of course, very basic reasons as to why it is needed!

Educational changes
Organisational instability
Increased demand on nurse services
More litigious society
Isolation of many practitioners
Inadequate resources
Poor job satisfaction
Staff burn-out.

Box 1.1 Key issues.

Accountability, Peer Review and Empowerment

The nurses' Code of Professional Conduct (UKCC, 1984) emphasised the importance of professional accountability, but in the 1990s the educational and organisational changes combined with higher public expectations from their health services made all health care staff more vulnerable in an increasingly litigious society. Today, in the United Kingdom all healthcare professional regulators are subject to the terms of the United Kingdom Council of Healthcare Regulators. This Council aims to ensure that each regulatory body works according to principles of public protection. Healthcare regulators are also active in *defining* the individual professions within healthcare, controlling entry to them, setting standards of conduct and imposing sanctions on individual professionals whose practice falls below these standards. Each practitioner is accountable to their own regulatory body for their standard of professional practice and to the employer for working within mutually agreed parameters. In her excellent paper, Cowie (2005; p. 33) discussed the dynamic effects on nursing brought about by a changing health service, saying that:

> The regulatory framework within which health care professionals operate exists to protect the public to whom professionals provide a service. In taking on new work, both employers and practitioners must assure themselves that the work can be performed in a safe and skilled manner. This is a basic pre-condition to ensure public protection. It requires that practitioners acknowledge any limits in their competence and decline duties until that competence has been achieved. Employers are required to ensure

that local policies are compatible with professional regulatory principles and that practitioners who expand their practice, or who participate in the development of new or modern roles, are facilitated to achieve the skills and competencies they need. Employees, in return, must work in accordance with their agreed role description.

The pressure on nurse practitioners to meet professional and public expectations is tremendous. Given these multiple impacts some mechanism was, and still is, needed to fill the many voids in working conditions for nurses. As Handy (1994; p. 2) remarked:

> if ... progress means that we have become anonymous cogs in some great machine, progress is an empty promise.

And progress, or reaching our potential, was and remains the big drive in nursing.

Nursing development units have shown the way to develop nurse-led services; advances in anaesthesia and surgery have changed the face of traditional surgical care from lengthy inpatient times to day surgery, and the altered focus of care from the acute sector (hospitals) to the community has meant that there is much that the nursing profession can own – indeed at times it seemed we can do anything and everything! We have gone beyond 'coping' and now instigate change, sometimes giving little thought to whom, if anyone, will pick up the work we have abandoned in our desire to 'progress'. Less notice has been given to the notion voiced by Dickson and Pickersgill, the main authors of a working document for the Nursing Directorate (NHSE, 1992), who while stressing the belief in a wealth of untapped potential in the nursing workforce, stated:

> Neither nursing nor any of the health disciplines are ends in themselves and the task facing the health service must be to ensure that staff are able to do everything possible to maximise patient well-being not only by improving the care received by every individual ... but also by ensuring that professionals and other staff are empowered ....

The major thrust to bring support to staff, as a process of empowerment, began by the formal introduction of clinical supervision onto the wider nursing agenda in the early 1990s, led by the Nursing Division at the DoH. Almost all initiatives deriving from the government attracts a degree of cynicism, often wholly justified, not least because funding is rarely attached to the dictats. However, a combination of events related to poor practices and overstressed nurses crystallised the need for some mechanism to support safe accountable practice. The demands on nurses to be innovative, to develop new skills and to be answerable for their actions and constantly update their knowledge were initially highlighted in the UKCC guidelines for professional accountability (UKCC, 1992) which stated that the practitioner

> must act in a manner so as to promote and safeguard the interests and well–being of patients and clients, maintain and improve professional knowledge and competence.

The Patient's Charter (DoH, 1991) and the Named Nurse Initiative within that Charter which promised a named qualified nurse, midwife or health visitor to every patient put further pressure on an under-resourced workforce. While the inclusion of a qualified nurse for every patient in the Act was welcome to the profession, the implications were considerable. In the event, the Named Nurse Initiative often fell well below the letter of the initiative, let alone the spirit! This was disheartening to a well-educated profession that had such high hopes of bringing the best of nursing care to patients. The Patient's Charter (NHSE 1991) was abolished as part of the changes to the NHS implemented in 2000 under the NHS plan (DoH, 2000), which promoted, among other changes, the extended roles of nurses and therapists – no reduction in challenge here then!

Nursing across the board has only seriously considered the value of supervision in meeting challenges since the 1990s, and I suspect that much of the reluctance to embrace it derived from a distaste for the system of managerial supervision used by some colleagues in other disciplines in the health services. For example the British Association of Counsellors (BAC), within their first Code of Ethics (BAC, 1984) made supervision mandatory for those in practice. Midwifery supervision is also a mandatory requirement for all practising midwives; it is responsible for monitoring and regulating their work, and in ensuring public protection. However, the difference between clinical supervision and management supervision was emphasised, ironically, by the UKCC (2001) advocating that midwives should consider accessing clinical supervision *in addition* to their statutory supervision. In nursing there are other mechanisms to provide management interventions and assessments – clinical supervision is *not* about that. Let's be very clear about what clinical supervision is not! It is not psychotherapy or counselling, nor is it a management tool or part of any performance review system. As Swain pointed out (1995; p. 16) it is '… **not** a form of disciplinary procedure'.

Nursing does not have a history of peer review; that is, a culture of self-critique and collegiate challenge, except when an individual or team submits an article or paper for publication in a quality journal. Getting published is not the aim of the majority of nurses, so the opportunity to obtain external or impartial expert advise in nursing is less than, for example, in medical specialities, or in academia, where it is common practice to present one's work to colleagues and to have it viewed and discussed analytically. Learning to critique and value other people's work in a constructive way is not easy, and requires a great deal of tact and honesty. However, learning to give and to receive comments on one's work is the professional fertiliser for growth and confidence. When you consider the delicacy, the intimacy, the technical and manual effort that goes into nursing it is insane not to develop a mechanism to nurture practitioners! The results of a Delphi study commissioned by the DoH (Butterworth and Bishop, 1995) on what facilitated good practice indicated that practitioners rated clinical supervision very highly as an empowering and stress-reducing mechanism. This parity of professional and government opinion was further developed in the new DoH nursing and midwifery strategy, which was spearheaded by the author. The new Vision for the Future: The nursing, midwifery and health visiting contribution to health and health care (DoH, 1993) had specific targets, of which clinical supervision was one.

Clinical Supervision: So What Is It?

First – What It Isn't!

The word 'supervision' smacks of 'overseeing' and both tend to have their roots in managerial command – strongly hierarchical and not sympathetic to the individual who is being overseen! Moving from this somewhat Dickensian approach to workers we have the artisan approach to learning, the apprenticeship model. This model is usually applied to those involved in a craft or area of expertise which is learned over a period of time, maybe years, such as building, carpentry, fine arts and the like. The process of 'learning through doing', is based on the novice watching, asking questions, and practising. It is interesting to remember that many of the early nurses were untrained nuns, novices in a fiercely hierarchical environment, and until a few decades ago nurse training in the United Kingdom, and in many other countries, had blended the vocational aspects of caring derived from religious orders with the apprenticeship model of skilled artisans. There is, however, an assumption here that the expert is absolute in their expertise, which does not fit the concept of lifelong learning – a concept held dear in nursing today, and essential with fast changing technologies and interventions. Within the health professions clinical supervision has offered a way of moving from a position of hierarchical authoritarianism to professional ownership of standards. This powerful mechanism has not been grasped eagerly, and one may wonder why? One reason may be that the concept has not been sufficiently explained to practitioners, many of whom regard it as a time consuming nuisance and unnecessary, and hopefully this book will go some way to addressing that. Another is certainly the lack of resources to implement it properly, which may not just be a financial argument but also an issue of control.

Names or titles are tricky – the term 'supervision' we have agreed, is a poor one to describe the process intended as it has connotations of task-oriented authority, and control by another. Nursing already had 'preceptorship' and 'mentorship' for newly qualified and less experienced nurses. So what is so different about clinical supervision, and why would a qualified person need to be supervised? Surely that would undermine the transition of nurse education into higher education, and the concept of an autonomous practitioner? Given that the term 'mentorship', which might have fitted the bill better, had already been assigned to a similar but different task, and added to which the term clinical supervision had already long been accepted by other therapists and mental health nurses, we were somewhat stuck with it.

Clinical Supervision: What It Is

Butterworth and Faugier (1992) traced the term clinical supervision to those professions with a history of it as a way of working, and where its utility and usefulness were not questioned. Rather, it is seen to have an inherent value which has become part of a working doctrine. We have noted that many mental health nurses have a longstanding knowledge of clinical supervision but the concept has been slow to filter into general nursing. The notion of reflective practice that allows practitioners, who are geared to rushing through a day's work in an attempt to meet all demands placed on them, to pause – ... ... consider their work away from the rush and thrust – is alien to many. Perhaps taking that time out to review and recall one's work may sometimes be painful, and using lack of time not to do so, can be an avoidance technique. Looking back on my clinical nursing, my most stressful time was when I was working in cardio-thoracic units. I can see now that I emotionally 'hid' behind the machines which I very efficiently managed, charted and even sometimes mended! It was a comparatively new time in that speciality, and patients often fared badly. Being efficient, and apparently 'coping so well' I was given more critical patients than any other nurses on the unit. No surprise that I suffered 'burn out'! Clinical supervision would have offered, if not solutions, at least opportunities for expression of the many issues around facing death almost daily.

There appear to be two fundamental elements to clinical supervision that have been widely accepted within nursing. First, that it is regular protected time for facilitated reflection on clinical practice (Bond and Holland, 1998; Johns and McCormack, 1998) and second that it aims to help the individual practitioner to develop their skills (Butterworth, 1992; Bishop, 1998). Notwithstanding this general agreement within the literature regarding a common process and purpose of clinical supervision, there remains much misunderstanding and misinterpretation among nurses as to what it actually is (White et al., 1998). Greenwood (2001) noted that this is possibly further compounded by the potential conflict experienced when clinical supervision is used to maintain and develop professional and clinical standards, or is fuelled by occasional inclusion of personal therapy. Northcott (1996) considered the scepticism held by some nurses as understandable when within supervision for their personal development there may be scope for managerial control. However, I well remember chairing a conference at which Nigel spoke passionately on its value, finishing by saying – 'why are you sitting here talking about it? Get on and do it!'

Finding a definition of clinical supervision has both enriched and confused the growing body of knowledge that is developing on the subject. A definition was needed that would espouse individual and professional growth and support, as well as reflection on working relationships at personal and organisational levels. Individual and professional relationships cannot be separated here – professional growth presumes a personal ability to examine oneself and one's responses to working relationships. I have always said that we should focus on the two words within the one, 'super' and 'vision', for they really underline what we are striving for (Bishop, 1994; p. 35). In considering the supportive roles of mentorship and preceptorship it is essential to be accessible, responsive to others, trusted, comfortable with one's own abilities and respectful of others, a view supported strongly by Driscoll (2000). These form the basis of mentoring relationships, and are also integral to clinical supervision.

That nurses at all levels require a relationship that focuses primarily on the process and experience of nursing is, as Faugier, pointed out (Butterworth and Faugier, 1992) something the profession has been slow to accept – here we are over a decade later endeavouring to change a long-established culture of non-support. Nursing has, wrote a perceptive Faugier, traditionally been intolerant and suspicious of anything which smacks of indulgence, and effectively deals with such developments by regarding those participating as elitist (p. 19). What perhaps is most important with regard to the semantics is the use of the word 'clinical' – the focus is on clinical practice, the heart of what nursing is about. In an earlier publication (Bishop, 1998), I held the view, and still do, that the terminology must focus on clinical practice and support the best possible standards of care, but I do accept that there may be confusion with some definitions in the apparent endorsement of a managerial context, which hopefully this book will rectify. Power (1999; p. 29) categorically stated that in his view if clinical supervision is to work it should not be allowed to become:

- a management activity allowing for the overseeing of subordinates
- linked to the disciplinary process
- exclusively concerned with time-keeping, ranges of pay, hours of duty and rostering
- about having the supervisee's work controlled, directed or managerially evaluated
- a punitive or gratuitously negative experience for the supervisee

- a continuous discussion of mistakes, failings or errors on the part of the supervisee, without being balanced by a discussion of the supervisee's professional strengths and the positive aspects of his work.

It is undoubtedly this lack of differentiation between managerial and clinical supervision that has hindered many in taking clinical supervision forward. Interestingly, there are many who advocate the use of clinical supervision for management personnel – I have absolutely no argument with that, but my main focus in this book is on those with direct contact with patients and clients.

Definitions

I am supported in my view that clinical supervision must have at its centre a clinical focus by Butterworth, who with Faugier, devised this definition that was commonly used in the early days of introduction (Faugier and Butterworth, 1994):

> Clinical supervision is an exchange between practising professionals to enable the development of professional skills, an opportunity to sustain and develop professional practice.

The DoH (1993) in the Vision for Nursing document elaborated on this much used but somewhat succinct explanation to read thus:

> A term used to describe a formal process of professional support and learning which enables practitioners to develop knowledge and competence, assume responsibility and the safety of care in complex clinical situations. It is central to the process of learning and to the expansion of the scope of practice and should be seen as the means for encouraging self-assessment and analytic and reflective skills.

While many of the principles of clinical supervision are obviously encased here, the definition does not allow for designated and protected time, and the emphasis on safety of care in complex situations could be interpreted as excluding the apparently more mundane aspects of nursing. In Northern Ireland the Northern Health and Social Services Board established a working group of senior nurses who met to discuss the implementation of clinical supervision and defined it as:

> A practice focused, professional relationship to ensure high quality nursing practice and care to patients and to provide support to staff in their professional role. (NHSSB, 1998; p. 2)

The Nursing and Midwifery Council (NMC) assumed its statutory responsibilities from the UKCC as the regulatory body for nursing and midwifery on 1st April 2002, inheriting from the UKCC the standards already set by them until such time as new ones were determined. It also inherits from the now defunct English National Board for Nursing, Midwifery and Health Visiting (ENB), the responsibility to approve educational institutions and programmes leading to registerable or recordable qualifications. The NMC defines clinical supervision as:

> A practice focused professional relationship that enables you to reflect on your practice with the support of a skilled supervisor. Through reflection you can further develop your skills, knowledge and enhance your understanding of your own practice. (NMC, 2005)

While supportive of clinical supervision and cognisant of its important role in clinical governance, the NMC has done little to progress its implementation, stating 'that clinical supervision is best developed at a local level in accordance with local needs' (NMC website).

My preferred definition of clinical supervision as it is intended within the nursing professions is at the beginning of this chapter, and was initially formulated by a group of senior clinical practitioners in workshops that I facilitated in the South East of England through Anglia Polytechnic University. Those nurses were ahead of their time and showed a keen understanding of what was involved in this key concept – I enjoyed them enormously, challenging though they were, and as a consequence I have upheld and adopted our shared definition. However, very recently, I was working with some prison health care staff and while they approved of this definition they felt that there was a lack of practitioner focus, so the final line, I think, amends that perfectly, and the officer who provided it is gratefully acknowledged.

> Clinical supervision is a designated interaction between two or more practitioners within a safe and supportive environment,

that enables a continuum of reflective, critical analysis of care, to ensure quality patient services, and the well-being of the practitioner. (Bishop and Sweeny, 2006)

This may not slip from the tongue lightly but it embraces the tenets of clinical supervision, and in particular, indicates that clinical supervision is *not* a 'one stop shop' (Rafferty and Coleman, 2001; p. 93) but a career-long journey.

Organisational Issues

Clinical Governance

Clinical governance is primarily concerned with standards and with the dissemination of best evidence. The term 'governance' aims to ensure accountability and excellence in the corporate and the financial management of the NHS by focusing control locally. That clinical governance is an extension of financial governance to clinical practices is well described by Scott (2001) who emphasised that it is a concept that requires a considerable change in the culture of health carers. The need for organisations to provide effective, quality health care has been the subject of a number of policy and strategy documents in the United Kingdom within both the NHS and the independent sector. Several national and international initiatives have been developed to facilitate clinical governance, which focus on implementation of evidence-based practice (EBP), including the establishment in the United Kingdom of the National Institute for Clinical Effectiveness (NICE). The government document 'A First Class Service – quality in the New NHS' (DoH, 1998) stated that one of the key strategies for achieving quality was the introduction of clinical governance. Scott (2001; p. 38) noted:

> . . . considering the focus in healthcare in recent years has been on the financial agenda and managerial framework, we are presented with a challenge that demands a radical change in thinking, which will in essence require a fundamental change in culture.

Perhaps the most important principle of clinical governance is a commitment to high quality, safe, patient-centred services in clinical practice. The guru of quality since the 1960s, Donabedian, described the seven pillars of quality (Donabedian, 1990):

- Efficacy
- Effectiveness
- Optimality
- Acceptability
- Legitimacy
- Equity.
- Efficiency

While Donabedian acknowledged the equal importance of processes as well as outcomes, the drive to implement clinical governance has rarely allowed for tacit knowledge, or for some of the highly individual skills which nurses may develop out of empathy and therapeutic intent. So the slant of the original work has shifted in my view, moving from quality to EBP, which are not necessarily one and the same. Models used in clinical governance tend to have emerged from the work of a late chief medical officer and a regional public health director (Scally and Donaldson, 1998), which work well for care interventions that are clearly defined and measurable, but are less sensitive to many of the interventions and interactions carried out by nurses. Integral to clinical governance is patient satisfaction, which is an area that nursing can and should influence.

Clinical governance is something which nursing as a whole appears to embrace but I am not convinced that the profession really understands its role within this framework, and most importantly, how to maximise its effectiveness. We are apt, in nursing, to take on new concepts somewhat blindly, with the desire to show our willingness and adaptability overriding our usual common sense and questioning approach. Perhaps this is our recent heritage from buying into a management culture rather than a patient-centred one? Be that as it may, in the United Kingdom the concept of clinical governance has been developed to 'ensure excellence in care' and while there are variations in standards that challenge both policy makers and managers, as well as clinical staff, the framework (at least the semantics for it) is in place. How it is developed depends on different organisations and their commitment, as well as government drivers. Scott (1999; p. 173) stated that, to be successful:

> ...the clinical governance agenda must be aimed at all professional groups and individuals and therefore a framework which reflects clinical development and activity is essential.

She added that the success of a clinical governance framework would depend on the ability of health care professionals to inform and influence each other – a key component of clinical supervision. Scott acknowledged that while the theory of clinical governance is easy the application is difficult. She charged nurses to be aware of their integral role and to identify the competencies and skills needed to enhance their influence and work as equal partners in decision-making processes.

Such professional confidence does not develop overnight, and without strategies in place to support professional development such as clinical supervision, nurses are less likely to feel sufficiently supported to present as equal with more dominant disciplines. Participating in clinical supervision in an active way within the context of an overall framework, rather than as a personal and isolated activity, is a clear demonstration of an individual exercising their responsibility under clinical governance. The cultural changes in the United Kingdom with increased personal responsibility are reflected in health care globally. There is a move from the paternalistic model of care, where the medical practitioner holds sway, to one where all health care professionals are required to demonstrate the effectiveness of their interventions. This means that systems need to be in place that allow service providers to measure the effectiveness of their care and to recognise where improvements are needed. The NHS is always a main focus of public concern, a political football being kicked high. Whatever government is in power the incumbents have to build to a great extent on existing structures, with of course, a snip here or a tuck there, to indicate change for the better! Currently in the government document 'A First Class Service – Quality in the new NHS', clinical governance is described as:

> A framework through which the NHS organisations are accountable for continuously improving the quality of their services and safeguarding high standards of *care by creating an environment in which excellence in clinical care will flourish.* (DoH, 1998; my emphasis)

This is a definition which, in the view of Professor Alan Maynard (1999) health economist and co-director of the York Health Policy Group, is practically useless, vague and circular. Despite the fact that most healthcare is delivered by teams, of which nurses are an essential part (Bloor and Maynard, 1998), Maynard noted that most of the evidence base is dominated by doctors. However, he considered that the challenges (and I would suggest opportunities) created for nurses by the development of clinical governance are considerable. His particular focus in the 1999 paper is related to nursing research, and he questioned our ability to enter the debate on clinical effectiveness when our evidence base has been (and still is) so poorly funded. This certainly makes a nonsense of the implied unity and equity of a governance framework, raising an ethical issue that nursing must address. Normand noted that within the concept of clinical governance there are always conflicting interests (Normand, 2004). The nursing profession needs to identify, unapologetically, its unique contribution to health care and clinical supervision is the ideal framework for that. Properly conducted it will ensure that standards are maintained, that interventions are appropriate, and that despite a frenetic pace of work, individual nurses can function therapeutically, rather than become mini bureaucrats distanced from the humanity of care.

The literature surrounding EBP originates in medicine and implies a strong orientation towards randomised controlled trials. This is sometimes in contradiction to nursing decisions which are often made in random and intuitive ways (Freshwater and Broughton, 2001; p. 67). Rafferty et al. (2004; p. 33) noted with regret the minimal reference to nursing and therapists in many of the strategic documents, a matter of some concern given the amount of time and care provided by them. As a profession we still have some way to go in gaining the confidence to promote our viewpoint in the delivery of care. Being 'on the job' for many years, keeping up to date with professional issues and development are only pieces in this ever-changing jigsaw called health care. As Rafferty et al. (2004; p. 35) stated, professional expertise is no longer sufficient guarantee of quality, and now an elaborate system of accountability and audit has developed to evaluate professional decision making. NHS priorities are set within National Service Frameworks, and service managers are hard pressed to meet centrally driven targets. Set against this management push was the professional pull for the nursing professions to take on new roles. These were emphasised in the document 'Making a Difference' (DoH, 1999), the strategic document for nursing, midwifery and health visiting, in which new or extended roles for nurses were advocated, in particular that of the consultant nurse. Hughes (2003; p. 1) summed up the situation neatly when he stated:

> Nurses working in Western health care at the start of the twenty-first century find themselves in a period of rapid change and sometimes turbulent organisational change. Often it is not clear whether this represents an opportunity for professional advancement or a threat to existent professional norms and working conditions.

If nursing is to survive as a practising, caring profession it must be used as an advantage for professional advancement.

> Clinical governance represents one of the strongest levers by which to persuade management of the necessity of clinical supervision – it is the touchstone of clinical standard setting

Management Commitment: Personal Development

Clinical supervision is not a camouflage to hide hierarchical domination. It is a mechanism to empower practitioners and requires time and investment. It is not, when properly carried out, a cheap option, but the benefits must be set against the advantages of safe, confident practitioners who are motivated and stable. High staff turnover and heavy litigation costs must be a penalty no organisation wants or can afford. As has been stated previously (Bishop, 1994) clinical supervision is not a substitute for poor management or a back door means of staff appraisal. To be effective it needs strong management commitment and funding for supervisees time and, at least, for supervisory training. While nurse executives to whom I have spoken are clear that nurses must own clinical supervision I sometimes had the feeling that this is an excuse not to facilitate its implementation. If an organisation is not proactive in any initiative the staff are unlikely to perceive it as a useful road to travel. Work by Kohner (1994) in her study of the DoH funded Nursing Development Units (NDUs), and Butterworth et al. (1996) in the multi-site study of clinical supervision identified similar organisational requirements that are essential for the successful implementation of clinical supervision. See Box 1.1.

- Management commitment at every level
- Protected resources in terms of budget, time, man-power and training
- Supervision for supervisors
- Establishment of evaluation techniques
- Application of evaluation data to service management

Box 1.2 Organisational requirements.

McSherry et al. (2002) argued that implementation of clinical supervision requires organisational support, both to raise awareness and to 'sell' it as a concept. Agenda for Change (DoH, 2005) requires a greater expectation that organisations provide a supportive environment whereby all staff can develop themselves and contribute to the development of others. Personal and people development is one of the core dimensions of all jobs covered by the NHS Knowledge and Skills Framework (KSF), which underpins the career and pay progression stand of Agenda for Change. Alongside other support measures such as appraisals and mentoring, clinical supervision is endorsed as a means of developing staff (DoH, 2004; 2005). Many practitioners are developing the skills of giving an account of practice, through the processes of reflective practice and through attending or taking part in research conferences at local, national and international level. Many nurses to whom I have spoken across the United Kingdom and who have taken part in clinical supervision say that they have developed an unexpected confidence – a bonus, if you like, over and above the expected support and professional exchange. They attribute this to taking time to examine their work and reflect with another experienced person; the sharing of knowledge and participation in agreed standards of care. The value of this interaction should not be underestimated, but neither should the courage it takes to enter into a challenging yet trusting relationship. Many practitioners have found that after participating in clinical supervision for a while they are far more active in the health care team in which they work, and are more likely to speak up rather than leave a meeting wishing that they had spoken their view if it did not coincide with more senior staff. The acceptance of one's own accountability is part and parcel of being a professional, as is audit of one's work. The framework of clinical supervision gives nurses the opportunity to reflect on their practice, identify shortcomings and build on strengths, and with the confidence gained, to take advantage of organisational changes to promote the quality of care in their clinical areas.

Conclusion

This chapter has explained the usefulness of clinical supervision, set within the policy pull and professional push of dynamic health care services. Its relationship to clinical governance is explored, with emphasis on the need to interact as equals on health care teams. The role of strong management support for successful implementation of clinical supervision is stressed.

References

BAC (1987) cited by Hawkins and Shohet 1989.41. Supervision in the helping professions. Open University Press, Milton Keynes.

Berwick D (2004) NHS Live Masterclass. http://www.doh.gov.uk

Bishop V (1994) Clinical supervision for an accountable profession. *Nursing Times* 90(39): 35–37.

Bishop V (1998) Clinical supervision: What is it? In: Bishop V (ed.) *Clinical Supervision in Practice: Some Questions, Answers and Guidelines.* Macmillan/NTResearch, Basingstoke.

Bloor K and Maynard A (1998) Rewarding healthcare teams: A way of aligning pay to performance and outcomes. *British Medical Journal*, 316: 7131.

Bond M and Holland S (1998) *Skills of Clinical Supervision for Nurses.* Oxford University Press, Buckingham.

Buchan J (2003) Challenges of recruiting and retaining: some thoughts for policy makers. *NTResearch*, 8(4): 291–292.

Buchan J (2004) Paper presented as keynote at Facing the Future: Our capacity to care, 2nd national convention, 28th June. Edinburgh International Conference Centre, SEHD/NHS, Scotland.

Butterworth T, (1992) Clinical supervision as an emerging idea in nursing In: Butterworth T and Faugier J (eds) *Clinical Supervision and Mentorship in Nursing.* Chapman and Hall, London.

Butterworth CA, Carson J, White E, Jeacock J, Clements A and Bishop V (1996) Its good to talk? The 23 site evaluation project of clinical supervision in England and Scotland. Manchester University, Manchester.

Butterworth T and Faugier J (1992) *Clinical Supervision and Mentorship in nursing.* Stanley Thornes (Publishers) Ltd, Cheltenham.

Butterworth T and Bishop V (1994) NHSE Clinical Supervision Conference Proceedings. NHSE, London.

Butterworth T and Bishop V (1995) Identifying the characteristics of optimum practice: Findings from a survey of practice experts in nursing, midwifery and health visiting. *Journal of Advanced Nursing*, 22: 24–32.

Cowie A (2005) The dynamic effect on nursing of a changing health service: A Scottish perspective. *Journal of Research in Nursing*, Sage Publications, London. pp. 27–44.

Davidson J (1998) Snapshots from Scotland. In: Bishop B (ed.) *Clinical Supervision in Practice; Some Questions, Answers and Guidelines*. Macmillan/NTResearch, Basingstoke.

Department of Health (1989) Working for Patients, cmm555. HMSO, London.

Department of Health (1993) Vision for the Future: The Nursing, Midwifery and Health Visiting Contribution to Health and Healthcare. HMSO, London.

Department of Health (1994) Working in Partnership: A Collaborative Approach to Care. Report of the Government Review of Mental Health Nursing. HMSO, London.

Department of Health (1994) Clinical Supervision for the Nursing and Health Visiting Professions. CNO Letter 94(5). HMSO, London.

Department of Health (1998) A First Class Service: Quality in the New NHS Leeds.

Department of Health (1999) Making a Difference: Strengthening the Nursing, Midwifery and Health Visiting Contribution to Health and Healthcare. London.

Department of Health (2000) *NHS Plan*. Department of Health, London.

Department of Health (2004) *The NHS Knowledge and Skills Framework (NHS KSF) and the Development Review Process*. Department of Health, London.

Department of Health (2005) *Agenda for Change: NHS Terms and Conditions of Service Handbook*. Department of Health, London.

Donabedian A (1990) The seven pillars of quality. *Archives of Pathology and Laboratory Medicine*, 114: 1115–1118.

Driscoll J (2000) *Practising Clinical Supervision. A Reflective Approach*. Balliere Tindall.RCN, Oxford.

Faugier J (1992) The supervisory relationship. In: Butterworth T and Faugier J (eds) *Clinical Supervision and Mentorship in Nursing*. Stanley Thornes, Cheltenham.

Faugier J and Butterwoth T (1994) Clinical Supervision: A Position Paper. Manchester University, Manchester.

Fowler J (1996) The organisation of clinical supervision within the nursing profession: A review of the literature. *Journal of Advanced Nursing*, 23: 471–478.

Freshwater D and Broughton R (2001) Research and evidence-based practice, In: Bishop V, Scott I (eds) *Challenges in Clinical Practice*. p. 67. Palgrave Macmillan. Basingstoke.

Grant A and Townend M. In press. Mental Health Practice. *Journal of Psychiatric and Mental Health Nursing*, Blackwell Publishing, Oxford.

Greenwood AD (2001) What factors influence the provision of and access to clinical supervision? Report to the Florence Nightingale Foundation, London.

Handy C (1994) *The Empty Raincoat*. Hutchinson, London.

Hughes D (2003) *Nursing and the Division of Labour in Healthcare*. p. 1. Palgrave Macmillan, Basingstoke.

Johns C (1998) Opening the doors of perception. In: Johns C and Freshwater D (eds) *Transforming Nursing Through Reflective Practice*. Ch. 1. Blackwell Science, Oxford.

Johns C and McCormack C (1998) Unfolding the conditions where the transformative potential of guided reflection (clinical supervision) might flourish or flounder. In: Johns C and Freshwater D (eds) *Transforming Nursing Through Reflective Practice*. Blackwell Science, Oxford.

Kohner N (1994) *Clinical Supervision in Practice*. Kings Fund Centre, London.

Maynard A (1999) Clinical governance: Commentary. The unavoidable economic challenges. *NTReserach* 4.3. p. 189. Emap Publications London.

McSherry R, Kell J and Pearce P (2002) Clinical supervision clinical governance. *Nursing Times*, 98(23): 30–32.

NHSE (1992) *A Working Document; Revitalising the Strategy for Nursing*. NHSE, London.

NHSE Patient's Charter (1991) NHS Executive, Leeds.

NHSSB (1998) Update of clinical suspervision in the NHSSB area. Unpublished report. P.2. Belfast, Northern Ireland Health I Board.

Normand C (2004) Commentary. Encouraging and not discouraging nursing research. *NTResearch*, 9(6).

Northcott N (1996) Supervise to grow. *Nursing Management*. 2(10): 18–19

Nursing and Midwifery Council (2005) Accessed from the web 30.3.2005.

Pearson A (1998) Excellence in care: Future dimensions for effective nursing. In NTR Symposium proceedings. *Nursing Times Research*, 3(1): 25–27.

Power S (1999) *Nursing Supervision; A Guide for Clinical Practice*. Sage, London.

Rafferty AM, Newell R and Traynor M (2004) Research and development: Policy and capacity building. p. 33. In: Freshwater D and Bishop V (eds) *Nursing Research in Context; Appreciation, Application and Professional Development*. Palgrave Macmillan, Basingstoke.

Rafferty M and Coleman M (2001) Developmental transitions towards effective education preparation for clinical supervision. In: Cutliffe J, Butterworth T and Proctor B (eds) *Fundamental Themes in Clinical Supervision*. Routledge, London.

Scally G and Donaldson LJ (1998) Clinical governance and the drive for quality improvement in the new NHS in England. *British Medical Journal*, 317: 61–65.

Scott I (1999) An opportunity for nurses to influence the future of healthcare development. *NTResearch*, 4(3): 170–175.

Scott I (2001) Clinical governance: A framework and models for practice. In: Bishop V and Scott I (eds) *Challenges in Clinical Practice*. Palgrave Macmillan, Basingstoke.

Swain G (1995) *Clinical Supervision: the Principles and Process*. p. 16. Community Practitioners and Health Visitors Association, London.

UKCC (1984) Code of Professional Conduct for the Nurse, Midwife and Health Visitor. UKCC, London.

UKCC (1986) Project 2000: A New Preparation for Practice. UKCC, London.

UKCC (1992) The Scope of Professional Practice. UKCC, London.

UKCC (2001) Supporting Nurses and Midwives Through Lifelong Learning. UKCC, London.

Webster C (2002) *The National Health Service. A Political History*. Oxford Press, Oxford.

White E, Butterworth T, Bishop V, Carson J, Jeacock J and Clements A (1998) Clinical supervision: Insider reports of a private world. *Journal of Advanced Nursing*, 28(1): 185–192.

Woods D (1992) The therapeutic use of self. In: Butterworth T and Faugier J (eds) *Clinical Supervision and Mentorship in Nursing*. Stanley Thrones (Publishers) Ltd.

2

Clinical Supervision: Functions and Goals

Veronica Bishop

SYNOPSIS

In this chapter, the functions of clinical supervision are discussed and the various models used are identified. A convergence model that sits within clinical governance is proposed. The need to use oneself and be open to self-development and critique in an environment of trust is stressed.

Introduction

It is important to state firmly at the outset of this chapter that clinical supervision is not something that 'gets done' to people. When considering the following text do not read it as a one-way system – a senior advising a junior. Rather see it as processes that all practitioners can give and receive, as long as they share an understanding of the intended goals.

Examining the different functions of supervision throws up various questions and issues, as Smith pointed out in his excellent paper on the function of supervision (1996). He asked 'in whose interest does supervision work?' The answer to this is somewhat circular. I hope that in Chapter 1 I have raised very comprehensive reasons for the inclusion of clinical supervision in any area of care where the clinicians are face to face with patients and clients. So, to answer Smith's question I would respond that the *users* of a health care system are the beneficiaries in the long term, with a more caring and better educated workforce interacting with them. In tracing the move of clinical supervision from psychotherapy to other health care professions, and its gradual concentration on the educational and evaluative elements of the supervisory situation, Faugier (1992; p. 21) stated:

> Increasingly, supervision is being viewed as an essential educa-
> tional process vital to the acquisition of effective therapeutic
> skills, central to professional growth. Supervision is about the
> overall functioning of the therapist in the clinical situation ...

While she regretted that too often models of clinical supervision are transferred lock, stock and barrel with little reference to appropri-ateness, Faugier asserted that the primary task of supervision is to assist supervisees in gaining knowledge that is lacking, to help them establish and maintain therapeutic relationships, and to overcome resistance to learning. Put simply, without any challenge to your knowledge base, or to your presumptions on care delivery, how will you develop? How can you possibly know what you don't know? Woods (1992; p. 39) emphasised that all nursing activity takes place in the context of a human relationship, and as such it is important for nurses to recognise and value the uniqueness of this human rela-tionship. Down (2002; p. 40) wrote movingly of her experiences in a critical care setting and of how receiving clinical supervision has had a profound effect on her personal and professional life, saying that clinical supervision

> ... provid[es] a window through which to view my practice,
> highlighting the need to know myself in order to be of therapeu-
> tic use to the patient and their families.

She went on to say that the impact clinical supervision had on her was to transform her practice and to celebrate nursing as a therapy, 'to be cherished and nurtured'. I recall my own days in ITU – a spe-ciality that I loved, but I never had what Down described and I would have been so much better at my work if that opportunity had been there for me. I am jealous! Heron (2001) wrote of the grace, character and culture of people who help people, saying that they 'move by the grace within the human spirit'. He considered that this grace is entirely independent of professional training, which can inform and enhance it or, conversely, obscure, suppress and distort it. It is certainly the bedrock of good nursing, and that must mean grace towards each other as well as to patients and clients.

- Emotional support, 'debriefing', nurturing
- A buffer mechanism
- Opportunity for critique from a peer or expert
- Professional development
- Time to reflect on one's work
- Trust

Box 2.1 Key issues: The functions of clinical supervision.

Functions of Clinical Supervision

The texts below are all interconnected, but for easy reference and quick reading, they have been separated into headings. Box 2.1 encompasses the key functions of clinical supervision.

Emotional Support

Serious illness, death and bereavement, child protection issues, abuse and disfigurement are some of the events that face many health care professionals. The emotional responses to these will vary, depending on the experience and attitudes of the individual practitioner. Stress may be felt at other times too – it is not always the dramatic event that triggers it off – inadequate facilities, poor staffing, a feeling of not being valued, any of these can lead to an emotional low. The concept of allowing work time to address the emotional needs of staff – referred to by Hawkins and Shohet (1989) as 'pit-head' time when miners washed the coal dust from their faces before going home – had been criticised by Yegdich (1999) and to a degree by Faugier (1992) who considered that the focus of clinical supervision should be on developing clinical practice rather than the personal needs of staff. While it is not suggested that this emotional support should be of a personal nature, it is important in the view of many that staff are nurtured during stressful times at work – what is often referred to as 'debriefing' in the forces and other sectors, such as emergency fire services, where stark events can shock or even traumatise the worker.

Woods (1992) emphasised the importance of nurses creating and maintaining therapeutic relationships that are going to be ultimately helpful in restoring patients to as healthy a position as possible, and suggested that if nurses are to achieve this they must make greater efforts to enhance the use of their feelings and emotions. Bond and Holland (1998) expressed this as:

> redressing a major imbalance in nursing education and practice which denies the power of emotions and the effect of hidden feelings in the way we relate to and communicate with others. (p. 67)

The use of self here is important, for it not only marks the shedding of traditional cool and possibly unfeeling efficiency behind the uniform, but denotes an understanding of self which can be usefully transferred in relationships with patients. This can be a risky business – we may presume an understanding that is not there; people mask their inner feelings, particularly if they are not in control of their environment. Discussion with a more experienced person, in complete safety, offers the opportunity to explore possible interpretations that you may not have previously considered. An example of a mistaken interpretation occurred during my clinical work for my Ph.D. thesis. I explored, through qualitative and quantitative measures, the relationship between surgical patients' fear of surgery and of anaesthesia (Bishop, 1986) and vividly recall a lady in her twenties due to undergo relatively minor surgery, sitting on her bed, chatting brightly to her neighbours. I asked the nurse in charge how anxious she thought this patient was on a scale of 1 to 10. 'Oh, her – she's fine, no anxiety at all. She understands the procedure and is very got together', was the reply. My instruments told a very different tale and I was convinced they must be wrong. I mentioned to the lady my puzzlement that the measurements obtained were very different from her outward appearances. Instantly, her muscles visibly sagged and the façade was gone. Her aunt had died under an anaesthetic just a month or so before, and she was terrified! If the nurse who had judged this patient to be 'very got together' had been more perceptive, more open to looking under the façade, would she have had the skills to cope with the reality of the patient's emotions? How often do we say to people, 'How are you – good?' A 'closed sentence', not allowing the option of a negative response. That would mean taking time, a commodity in short supply, and would possibly require the understanding and expressing of emotions not easily accessed or swiftly repackaged! Good implementation of clinical supervision will allow you, the supervisee, time to express your anxieties in relation to work, to unpick your biases and to recharge your emotional battery.

Clinical supervision, if it had been available to me, would have saved me much emotional trauma. I will share with you a classic example: As a qualified general nurse working in an acute psychiatric unit for wider experience, I was told to shadow a patient who had attempted suicide by throwing herself under a tube train. She was, before the train lines burnt one side of her, a very attractive woman who was now at the very bottom of her personal hell. It was stressed as imperative that I never, at any time, left her alone – even the loo chain could spell disaster! Then the unit staff forgot about me. I was left on a one-to-one basis with this lady for days, until my attempts to be sympathetic and to strive for empathy rendered me fit to jump under the next train with her! While this is an extreme example of bad staff management, it must be remembered that nurses are not super human with all emotional baggage unpacked and neatly shelved.

Of course family and friends may provide much of this support, but without an understanding of the professional issues involved it is unlikely that they could offer the knowledgeable challenge that may be useful to a practitioner, or be sufficiently detached to critique honestly. However, within this professional approach to critique must be a regard from the supervisor to the supervisee, an appreciation of what they have achieved and their potential for more Freshwater (2002) considered that every conception of self is conceived of as a by-product of the relationship between power and knowledge, and she defines self-esteem as the evaluative aspect of the self. The need to feel that one has some control over one's life is equally important in any work situation, and a very influential aspect of a person's approach to their practice. The apathy that may accompany the supervisee who has perhaps suffered one too many organisational change, or who feels that they are just a cog in a wheel, will present quite a challenge to the most committed supervisor. Similarly, so will the real or perceived discrepancy between the demands of work and the resources available. This does not mean that anyone who is not a wizard at refreshing the downhearted, burnt out or complacent should not learn to be a supervisor – though such magic would be welcome – but it does mean that supervisors must expect to be a buffer between some of the harsh reality and the practitioner.

The New Oxford dictionary (1998) defines a buffer as a person or thing that prevents incompatible or antagonistic people or things from coming into contact with or harming each other. In clinical supervision this is not enough – a resolution to the antagonism or incompatibility needs to be identified, so any model of clinical supervision must aim at facilitating emotion-focused coping as well as problem-focused coping. To achieve this the use of reflection and reflexivity is an invaluable resource, and is discussed further by Freshwater in Chapter 3. Offering care and empathy may at times carry a high cost, and the need to reflect, to recuperate, and possibly to admit one's own need for external counselling, can be recognised with skilled supervision. This is unlikely to happen without a great deal of trust in the supervisory relationship. Nurses may walk an emotional minefield every day, and while this is a very privileged position it is an exhausting one.

Critique

Increasingly, nursing is incorporating less traditional approaches to care such as aromatherapy and massage techniques, which have increased the opportunity and concomitant necessity for a sensitive therapeutic relationship between patients and nurses, and as such, the need for practitioners to reflect on their communications skills, and their intervention and evaluation processes. The need to understand and absorb new technologies and to meet the requirements of evidence-based practice is a constant challenge, particularly so for many practitioners who are quite isolated from their peers, and have scant opportunity for collegiate support and critique. Even for those practitioners surrounded by their peers, in the daily rush and thrust of a busy schedule we can, as Pearson (1998) noted, achieve the desired outcome in terms of health status *in spite* of the nursing that we provide, even if the nursing we provide dehumanises or devalues people. If we are to provide excellence in nursing we must consider how to support and acknowledge that excellence.

While clinical supervision is essentially a supportive mechanism, that support should not imply 'comfort zone'! Walsh et al. (2003) found in their evaluation of a model of clinical supervision that the group being studied, in its anxiety to be supportive was not sufficiently challenging, thus compromising their ability to reflect upon and critique practice. Being open to challenge is central to moving on, to building on the best and to ditching the inferior. Clinical supervision should challenge your actions, not always a comfortable situation, but one where it is important not to become defensive. Bond and Holland (1998; p. 93) observed that most nurses who receive training in supervisee skills need help with dealing with criticism, often from a misunderstanding as to the real intent of clinical supervision. Because nursing, even today, holds a very hierarchical view of the world, not helped by the term 'supervision', its members are apt to regard critique or questioning as a negative against them. Sometimes it may be the way you respond, for example, if you become aggressive or truculent, indicating that you don't wish to accept the criticism but know it to be true. Careful communication is important in any aspect of health care, and taking time to consider words and phrases may benefit not only the session but dealings with others too.

Critical debate about practice activity is a means to professional development and Butterworth (1992; p. 12) pointed a finger at nurses for not 'indulging' in critical debate as a matter of routine, suggesting that it stems from the minor input nurses make at ward rounds. I can remember when I was a student nurse on an orthopaedic ward that nurses, except for the Sister, were firmly excluded from one consultant's rounds – we were well and truly to be kept below stairs in his book! If there ever was any place for that kind of insular arrogance there certainly isn't now! Team working is central to health care services, and that means that each team member has an inherent responsibility to both give and receive feedback on their effectiveness within that team. Everyone has something to learn, and usually there is something that each player brings to the stage. Wilkin (1998; p. 194) acknowledged that constructive criticism is a crucial component of the supervisory process – as he put it:

> ... it is a necessary yet delicate art which every supervisor needs to employ in order to enable and empower the [practitioner]. If [they] are not challenged and encouraged to reflect on their practice, their blind spots will remain unseen and their development severely restricted ... Contrary to what some people believe, criticism can be positive and non-punitive.

He added that it may be an indicator of a person's maturity if they feel unable to accept confrontation that is offered within a nurturing framework. Certainly a degree of maturity is needed to move to the situation described by Todd (2002) where the supervisory process has led to the development of an 'internal supervisor'. This is achieved when the supervisee develops the capacity for spontaneous reflection-in-action; moving from retrospective reflection to awareness of one's thoughts and reactions to any given situation of the moment.

Mallik (1998) on her study tour to Australia, supported by the Florence Nightingale Foundation, used an illuminative case study approach to evaluate the role of nurse educators in the development of reflective practitioners with particular focus on clinical supervision. She noted that while in that country reflective practice is a domain that requires competence for registration (a powerful endorsement for its development) the actuality did not always match the curriculum documentation.

> An important part of critique is praise and encouragement. Examining others' work is an opportunity to examine one's own, and a good supervisor will 'reward' a supervisee by openly acknowledging where he or she had benefited from the session. Casement (1985) identifies being a supervisor as an endless opportunity to see our own errors and a chance to re-examine our own work.

Trust and Respect

The issues of trust and respect are import factors in the supervisory process, and it is appropriate here to mention the confusion that often arises in the early stages of implementation of clinical supervision, that is, the management function of the organisation. Lines of confidentiality must be clarified here. The UKCC, in the early stages of national implementation of clinical supervision, spent some considerable time debating the ownership of any information disclosed during a supervisory session. The Council concluded that while links between individual performance reviews will inevitably occur, any disclosure to management of information shared at a supervisory session should only occur at the request of the practitioner (Darley, 1995). The Nursing and Midwifery Council, which has replaced the UKCC, has not altered that approach. As has been stated before, it is unlikely that a supervisee will expose him or herself if there is not a complete trust that the exchange will be in confidence. It is important to note here, however, the words of

Dimmond, a lawyer and regular speaker at clinical supervision conferences, who wrote (2002; p. 28):

> It is not always appreciated that there is no right or privilege for a nurse, doctor or other health professional to respect the confidentiality of information provided by the patient when required to answer questions by a court of law. Even a priest would be legally bound to disclose information learnt in the confessional if the judge considered that information given by the confessor was relevant to an issue arising at court.

Similarly, any reflective diaries or notes made during work, or about work, could be called into court. Practitioners registered with the Nursing and Midwifery Council have a professional responsibility to raise any concerns relating to any circumstances in the environment of care, or where health and safety are at risk. All NHS organisations should have procedures within their management function that allow staff to report such incidences. These serious obligations aside, the supervisory interaction should be within an agreed contract between the parties involved, and should make clear that within the law, there should be no breach of confidentiality.

The trust that is implicit in clinical supervision is perhaps the hardest link in the chain to forge. Many practitioners to whom I have spoken have not developed a collegiate rapport or fellowship among their peers; I do not know if this is due to insecurity or competitiveness, poor management or a fairly mobile workforce that carries only a small burden of collegiate compassion and confidentiality towards their own! Whatever the reason it is counterproductive to achieving professional integrity and personal growth. However, trust has to be earned, and any supervisory relationship must, to be fruitful, be based on trust that not only matters discussed will be treated with utmost confidentiality but also on the supervisor's ability to critique knowledgeably. The importance of knowledgeable challenge and shared learning is central if clinical supervision is to play its rightful part in standard setting and clinical governance.

In the same way that trust is a two-way matter, so is respect. A supervisor should not be in a supervisory relationship with someone that they do not respect – nor should a supervisee be expected to share their vulnerability with a person they do not hold in high regard. Clinical supervision is not a one-way system.

Contracting: Legal Implications

Contracting

The relationship between the supervisor and the supervisee is at the centre of any model of clinical supervision used, and it is important to have clear guidelines or, preferably, an informal contract that states how the process is to be conducted. As Bond and Holland (1998; p. 201) acknowledged, anxieties not voiced about the supervisory relationship can negatively influence its implementation, and result in lack of rigour and support. Everitt (1996) described an example of a clinical supervision contract that takes into account the type of supervision agreed, its theoretical orientation and the boundaries and documentation of sessions, as well as issues of structure, confidentiality and (subjective) evaluation. The notion of a contract between supervisors and supervisees has been found to be helpful to many when getting started in clinical supervision, with clear working agreements laid out for supervisory relationships, and clarity of task and intent within the employing organisation. Further, it is crucial that there are clear and specific agreed boundaries of information and confidentiality between supervisor, practitioner and managers, as mentioned above. Contracts usually contain terms on frequency, duration, venue and format; that is, what kind, if any record is kept of the meetings, and who hold those records. have known good plans for implementation go to the wall for want of simplicity here! If notes are kept, keep them and their safe keeping clear and simple. Remember here the advise of Dimmond (2002; p. 28) regarding any notes or diaries regarding work – they may be, in peculiar circumstances, be demanded for use in legal cases.

> It is not always appreciated that there is no right or privilege for a nurse, doctor or other health professional to respect the confidentiality of information provided by the patient when required to answer by a court of law.

When setting up a contract it is useful to ensure that there is an agreement to review the effectiveness or suitability of the relationship after a given time – the 'get out clause' is essential for relationships that are either too cosy or too uncomfortable for either party. It is not humanly possible for everyone to feel at ease with everyone else – our diversity is what makes us such a rich professional

- Allocated time
- Regular meetings
- Choice of supervisor
- Mutual respect
- Agreed record keeping
- Confidentiality
- Agreed ground rules regarding access to supervisor
- Get out clause
- Feedback evaluation mechanism (see Chapters 5 and 7)

Box 2.2   Essentials for contracting in clinical supervision.

resource, and surely an example of professional maturity is the ability to discuss a relationship that may need changing. Box 2.2 highlights the essentials for a clinical supervision contract, and these need endorsement from the employing authority if implementation is to be successful.

Legal Implications

It is important to stress that clinical supervisors are not solutions people! The opinion of supervisors should never override that of the supervisee – any qualified practitioner is accountable for his or her own actions.

Giving advice should not be seen as the primary aim of clinical supervision. This may be difficult for many nurses to accept, as we are basically very practical people and seek solutions to problems so that we can move on – possibly to the next problem and the next if we don't work out why we are constantly hitting our head on a brick wall! *Remember – sometimes there are no solutions, only methods of coping with the dilemma.* The tendency for supervisors to give advice, as opposed to helping the practitioner to reflect and arrive at a solution, is a real one, and one which Dimmond addressed:

> . . . if inappropriate or negligent advice were given to the supervisee there would be a possibility that the supervisor could be

held liable. Also if harm befell the supervisee as a result of following this advice, he/she might seek compensation from the employer for the negligence of employees acting in course of employment (vicarious liability). (Dimmond, 1998; p. 487)

Another issue that participants at conferences and workshops have raised with me is that of 'whistle-blowing'. Each NHS organisation should have an established procedure to ensure that staff may alert senior management of failures within the organisation that could endanger health or safety, including clinical governance. The Health care Commission as a watchdog of standards within the NHS should also provide a mechanism to ensure that staff concerns regarding standards are investigated. With particular regard to nurses, midwives and health visitors registered with the Nursing and Midwifery Council, each has a professional responsibility to report to an appropriate person or authority concerns relating to health and safety. Other registered practitioners have similar arrangements with their professional bodies. In the rare event of a supervisor considering the need to report a supervisee for negligent or dangerous practice, the supervisee should first be informed of the intended breach of confidentiality, and allowed the opportunity to deal with the matter directly with the appropriate authority. While it is foolish to ignore such contingencies, it must be remembered that clinical supervision sessions are usually about far less overtly dramatic matters, and talk of legalities should not put anyone off entering into what is potentially a rewarding experience.

All of these elements described above: the questioning approach to care, the development of communications skills for both the supervisee and the supervisor, the knocking down of conventional paternalistic barriers in approaches to patients and indeed to other staff, can only truly be realised within an organisation that values excellence and its staff who provide it, and in an atmosphere of trust and respect. This respect has to start somewhere, and while clinical supervision is unlikely to blossom within an organisation that is hierarchical and prescriptive, pockets of flowering can occur within local clinical areas if those involved have a shared understanding of its goals and how to achieve them, and are really committed to its principles.

It will now be clear that any model of clinical supervision should contain elements that encourage professional critique combined with

• Empathy	Trust	Confidentiality
• Support	Buffer	Listening
• Reflection	Professional knowledge	Openness
• Critique	Skill sharing	Respect
• Willingness to learn	Communication skills	Commitment
• Challenge	Encouragement	Accountability
• Organisational support	Time	No blame culture

Box 2.3   Clinical supervision requirements for all parties: Supervisees, Supervisors and Organisations.

some emotional outlet and support. If this implies that supervisors have to be qualified therapists, consultants in their area of clinical work, and digest reams of up-to-date research on a daily basis – not true. Don't panic! Supervisors need to care, to have controlled empathy with their colleagues, and an understanding of the work that their supervisee undertakes. *Compassion and educated skill is what nursing is about* – any nurse can, if he or she is motivated to do so, become a supervisor to another nurse or colleague in their area of knowledge. The role of the supervisor is discussed far more fully in Chapter 4, but it is helpful to touch on it at this stage to place models of clinical supervision in context. So what are the basic requirements for any model of clinical supervision? Box 2.3 encapsulates these, but – and this is a big BUT – training is essential for all involved, both supervisees and supervisors (who in my view must also be supervised if still in practice) if this rich cocktail of personal and managerial requirements is to be successfully mixed and enjoyed.

Models of Clinical Supervision

In the proper search for appropriate models of clinical supervision it would 'be tragic if the generous and essential intentions of clinical supervision for the support of quality practice are lost as egocentric theoreticians develop and promote over-complex models which have less to do with utility and more to do with being labelled' (Butterworth et al., 1996; p. 128). A model described by Proctor (1986) was adopted, in the main, by UK Trust nurse executives, when early national discussions took place on clinical supervision. It was the model adapted by Faugier and Butterworth (1992), who built substantially on the emotional and caring components, stressing the need for a trusting relationship between supervisors and supervisees and the opportunity to bring a questioning approach to nurses, in a non-threatening environment. This model strongly focuses on growth and support, unsurprising given their mental health background, and was seen as highly suitable for general nurses whose training until recently, lacked any connection with the 'self'. The Proctor model has certainly provided the basis for many subsequent models and addresses what are termed formative (developmental and educational), normative (professional standard setting), and restorative (de-stressing, recharging) functions, and these are now described more fully.

Formative/Developmental/Educational

Hawkins and Shohet (1989; p. 42) express the learning thus:

- To understand the client better
- Become more aware of their own reactions and responses to client
- Understand the dynamics of how they and their client are interacting
- Look at how they intervened and the consequences of their interventions
- Explore other ways of working with this and other similar client situations.

What is intended within the context of the formative/educational element of clinical supervision is not an alternative to management objectives, it is the provision of a highly personal professional reflective space.

Walsh et al. (2003), in an Australian study devised for a community mental health nursing team, identified this element of clinical supervision as the educative process used in developing the knowledge and skills of the supervisee, achieved by sharing knowledge relevant to practice and through the enhancement of self-awareness. This focus on the educational aspect of clinical supervision does not in any way detract from knowledgeable support from others, such as tutors, ward managers or the like. On the contrary, it is complementary. For those solely concerned with clinical work action learning Revans (1976) believed that effective learning only really begins when people have the opportunity to constructively share their difficulties, concerns and experiences with others. It is certainly a method of learning that lends itself to the sharing of experiences that is intrinsic to the concept of clinical supervision. Learning at the time an event is taking place, while invaluable, can be a limited process. It is usually restricted to the actions and reactions of the event, rather like a framed photograph of a moment in time. It is when you take out the photograph later, and recall the events prior to it, and the sounds and colours that are held within it, that you can reflect more fully on its composition.

Taking the slightly compartmentalised Proctor model a stage further, and owing much to counselling, reflective learning has been developed (see Chapter 3) and recognised in nursing (see, for example, Johns, 1995; Rolfe, 1998; Freshwater, 2002) over the past decade. Johns perceived reflection to be a purposeful activity that is at the core of clinical supervision (2003). True to his philosophy of a 'reflective traveller' he constantly seeks better forms or definitions to describe the process. Preferring a description to a definition he stated that

> Reflection is being mindful of self, either within or after an experience, as if a window through which the practitioner can view and focus self within the context of a particular experience, in order to confront, understand and move forward toward resolving contradiction between one's vision and understanding .... (Johns, 2005; p. 2)

Johns developed a model for structured reflection (MSR) which constructs ways of knowing against reflective cues (Johns, 2004). Far from being prescriptive, he intended the model to be used in conjunction with reflexivity and suggested that sensible practitioners use such models creatively to suit themselves. Any model adopted or adapted must suit the values and philosophy of the individual to be meaningful. Kadushin (1992; p. 20), when writing of supervision in social work regarded the primary problem in supervision as ignorance of the supervisee regarding the skills and competencies to do the job; thus, a main objective of supervision is one of teaching. Given that in social work supervision is an overtly managerial function this comment is not directly transferable to nursing. Clinical supervision is not an educational stop gap, or as has been said before, a cover for poor management. However, we can concur with

Kadushin that supervisees may be helped to understand the client or patient better and that one of the primary goals is to upgrade skills, although I would add another is to nurture practitioners to enable the upgrading of skills.

Normative/Standard Setting

This function highlights the need for individual accountability and the setting of standards and competencies to achieve those standards. Van Ooijen (1996) developed a model – the normative functions model – that has some sympathies with the views of Kadushin. This was designed to take into account the necessary purchasing and contracting mechanisms of the internal market system used by the NHS at that time, but adapts well to today's clinical governance structure, see Figure 2.1.

This model highlights the routes by which to move from traditional positions of passive partnership to one of professional ownership of standards. This can be achieved by discussion of practices with experienced and knowledgeable colleagues who are able to identify examples of poor practice in a no-blame culture and make suggestions for changes and continuous improvement. There is the potential here for some overlap with organisational and management roles – however, clinical supervision is not, as has been

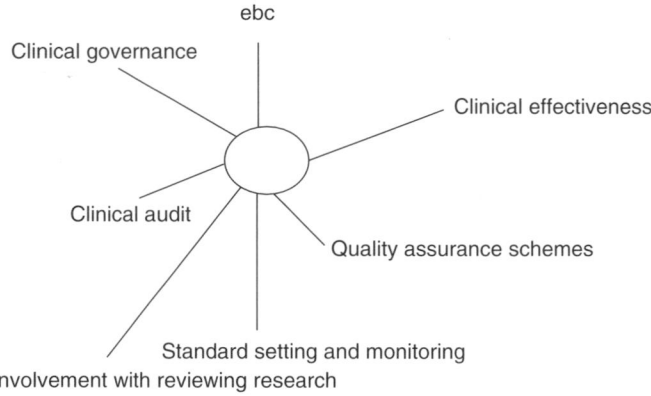

Figure 2.1   Normative functions of clinical supervision adapted from van Ooijen.

stressed before, a back door for management strategies, but has an obvious relationship with good practice and clinical governance. The relationship between the supervisee and supervisor is a working alliance, and must sit legitimately and securely within the shared working agenda with their organisation. Smith (1996; p. 5) remarked on managers' approaches to supervision and considered that it was the responsibility of any manager to monitor and improve the work of others. Pateman (1998; p. 178) supported the notion of management benefiting from the implementation of clinical supervision by giving examples of normative elements and linking them to professional and quality issues. For example, identifying the boundaries of one's role, working towards high standards, working within the code of professional guidelines and national legislation and local organisational policies. Added to this should be making links with research-based practice, and evidence-based practice networks; feeding into links with clinical governance. All this may sound daunting – but it need not be, with collegiate support and good management systems. Clinical supervision offers nursing and other health professionals the opportunity to move from traditional positions of passive partnership to one of professional ownership of standards.

Restorative: Support and Self-development

What happens to people when they experience high levels of stress over a long time, or feel that their input is not seen as of value? Apathy or a feeling of helplessness can result in people no longer striving to be effective, to meet their goals. Seligman (1975) described this as learned helplessness and considered it a principle characteristic of depression. Benner and Wrubel (1989) noted a number of unique sources of stress in nursing, including shift patterns of work, conflict between money-centred aims of management and the caring values of nursing, and the strong focus on clearly defined clinical outcomes that can deny nurses the opportunity to explore their unique contribution to health care. Personal control and health are seen to be related and an aim of clinical supervision must be to maintain or seek to regain the positive approach of a skilled workforce. Proctor (1986; p. 24) described the supportive function of clinical supervision as:

> . . . a way of supporting workers who are affected by the distress, pain and fragmentation of the client and how they need time to

become aware how this has affected them and to deal with reactions. This is essential if workers are not to become over full of emotions, or alternatively heavily defended against the distress of the client, therefore lacking empathy and good-enough care.

While a supportive and nurturing relationship for a novice practitioner is widely accepted in practice, the same cannot be said for staff who have been qualified for some time. Is this reasonable when healthcare changes too quickly, with new drugs, new technologies, new concepts? I doubt that there is anyone practising who is not regularly challenged in their thinking and would welcome (and benefit) from supported reflective time. Down (2002) noted how easy it is to lose sight of the humanness of patients, and reflected on the constant challenge to balance the art and science of nursing so that neither dominates. Challenging accepted practices, being involved in ethics and forging balanced relationships with other disciplines and staff is stressful in itself, without the natural distress of being with sick and often terminally ill people whom you are striving to care for with empathy. Bound in with this supportive component is the opportunity to consider one's own career, to take a moment of time to see yourself in the context of where you are and where you would like to be in career terms.

Expansion Models

Fowler (1996) expanded the Proctor model, proposing a framework with categories of intervention, to provide structure and purpose. Bond and Holland (1998) also advanced Proctor's model, emphasising that the means by which the normative function is addressed is through the medium of the restorative and supportive function. Whichever model or adaptation of a model is used in clinical supervision a key component must be that of giving support to the supervisee – that is, after all, its raison d'etre. Sarafino (2002; p. 105) altered the terminology from that used by Proctor, and identified five basic types of support, these being emotional/empathy, esteem/encouragement, tangible/direct assistance, informational/feedback and network/membership support, thus making more explicit the breadth of support to be offered to a supervisee. Certainly a good supervisor should endeavour to incorporate all or any of these, depending on the supervisee's needs at any one time.

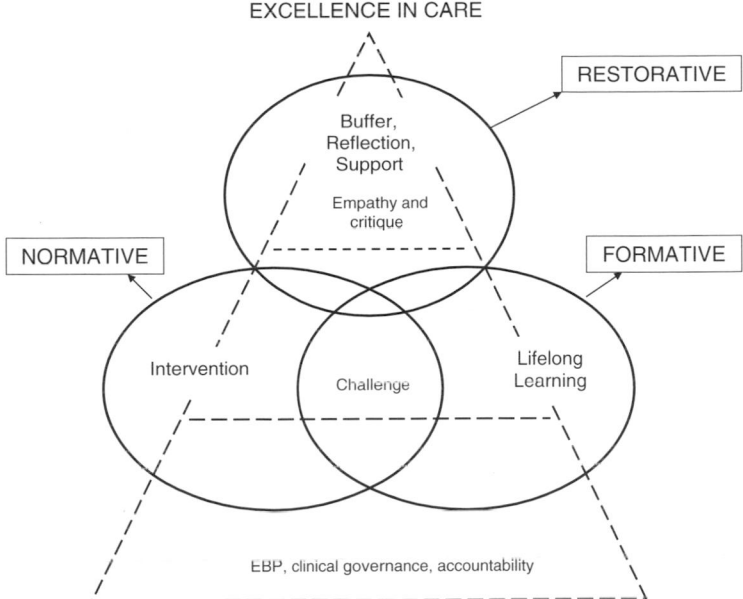

Figure 2.2   Convergence model of clinical supervision.

In bringing together Proctor's three-component model and Sarafino's more specific focus on support and professional development, the individual practitioner is potentially well nurtured. However, in the current (and I suspect long-term future, though the terminology may change) culture of clinical governance, there is no overt link between the individual and clinical governance that explicitly expresses the power of the practitioner to influence standards, and indeed, sit at the high table of the employing organisation. The model identified in Figure 2.2 is offered as an illustration of the convergence of the concepts described by Proctor and widened by Sarafino, and the influence of the individual participating in clinical supervision in the employing organisation. This convergence of theories and concepts places the practitioner firmly in the centre of the organisation while maintaining their personal cycle of professional development, and points to quality patient care. However, remember 'models' in themselves are no value unless they are used to guide a philosophy or plan of action; and the best ones are open to adjustment!

Convergence model of clinical supervision: clinical excellence

- Normative, formative and restorative functions
- Support/buffer mechanisms/empathy
- Reflection/feedback/critique/advice
- Challenge and intervention
- Clinical governance/standard setting/ebp/accountability.

Getting Going with Clinical Supervision

A constant complaint from people considering setting up a system of clinical supervision is that while there is a wide range of material on definitions, models and other surrounding issues, little exists to steer the novice organiser into getting clinical supervision up and running. It is not rocket science! All that is needed is organisational agreement (possibly the biggest hurdle), some consensus on how sessions are to be run, how often they are to be held and what, if any, notes are to be made of each session. A contract between an agreed supervisor and supervisee should be drawn up, which defines frequency of sessions, their duration and agreement to confidentiality within the terms of professional conduct. The Marie Curie Cancer Care (MCCC) implementation programme is a good example, and worth noting. A framework or strategy paper was drawn up by nurses, therapists and other staff and was disseminated across the hospices and community teams. The model selected was based on the Proctor model described in this chapter, and self-selected and invited experienced individuals were trained as supervisors in various localities. Supervision here is very multi-professional, and includes the chaplains as well as all clinically engaged staff. It is an opt-in policy rather than a mandatory one, but management are extremely supportive and facilitative to those involved in training and taking the concept forward. Individuals were limited by whom they may invite to be their supervisor owing to small staff numbers in each locality, but this is no longer the case with training for community nurses to be clinical supervision supervisors/facilitators. These staff receive their own supervision either in MCCC groups, or if they wish, outside the organisation. Sessions are generally held monthly, with all MCCC nurses and nurse managers able to access group supervision in work time. Occasionally, in the MCCC hospices one-to-one supervision is possible. It is planned to audit the policy by gathering quantitative information about the numbers of people receiving clinical supervision, cost, number of internal/ external supervisors, and to obtain data from supervisees regarding the perceived benefits from their sessions.

Interestingly, an online system is about to be piloted by MCCC, aimed at providing access to synchronous online clinical supervision for their community staff in the most rural areas. Should this mode of delivery prove to be successful it may be viewed as a method that can be added to the clinical supervision opportunities within the wider organisation.

Clinical supervision can be carried out in one of at least five ways. These typically are:

- One to one with an expert from your discipline
- One to one with an expert from another discipline
- One to one with a colleague of similar expertise
- Group supervision with colleagues working together
- Network supervision with people who do not usually work together.

The safety of one-to-one sessions may seem preferable initially, but as Johns noted (2003) individual supervision may limit developmental potential. Group sessions to be meaningful require skilled supervisors, but are more economic in terms of time and costs, and offer a wider perspective if sufficient trust is ensured. Jones (2003) found that group supervision was beneficial in her study of hospice staff but acknowledged that it may raise anxiety in all participants, and requires preparation and support for the facilitator. Today, with the benefits of web or email access electronic methods are being developed that will be of great help to those working in very rural and inaccessible areas such as the highlands of Scotland where I spoke to people who were travelling for five hours for a one-hour session! Issues such as security and confidentiality will need to be carefully addressed here, but there is no good reason why, carefully thought out, electronic access to supervision should not be a great success.

Conclusion

The diversity of approaches to implementing clinical supervision reflects the diversity of the stakeholders and the (still) developmental state of the activity. Whatever structure is used in clinical supervision the main aim of understanding interpersonal relations and progressing the delivery of care for patients and clients remains central.

References

Benner P and Wrubel J (1989) *The Primacy of Caring: Stress and Coping in Health and Illness*. Addison-/Wesley, Wokingham.

Bishop V (1986) The quantification of stress in patients immediately before and during anaesthesia and surgery. PhD thesis. London University. (RCN Steinberg Library).

Bond M and Holland S (1998) *Skills of Clinical Supervision for Nurses*. Oxford University Press, Buckingham.

Butterworth T (1992) Clinical supervision as an emerging idea in nursing. p. 12. In: Butterworth T and Faugier J (eds) *Clinical Supervision and Mentorship in Nursing*. Stanley Thornes (Publishers) Ltd., Cheltenham.

Butterworth T, Bishop V and Carson J (1996) First steps towards evaluating clinical supervision in nursing and health visiting. 1. Theory, policy and practice development. A review. *Journal of Clinical Nursing*, 5: 127–132.

Butterworth T and Faugier J (Eds) (1992) *Clinical Supervision and Mentorship in Nursing*. Chapman Hall, London.

Casement P (1985) *On Learning from the Patient*. Tavistock London, Cheltenham.

Darley M (1995) Clinical supervision and IPR. *Nursing Management*, 1:9.

Dimmond B (1998) Legal aspects of clinical supervision 2. Professional accountability. *British Journal of Nursing*, 7(8):487–489.

Dimmond B (2002) Legal aspects of patient confidentiality. *British Journal of Nursing Monograph*. Mark Allen Publishing Wiltshire.

Down J (2002) Therapeutic nursing and technology: Clinical supervision and reflective practice in a critical care setting. p. 40. In: Freshwater D. (ed.) *Therapeutic Nursing*. Sage, London.

Everitt J (1996) Stress and clinical supervision in mental health care. *Nursing Times*, 92(10): 34–35.

Faugier J (1992) Psychotherapy. p. 21. In: Butterworth T, Faugier J and Burnard P (eds) *Clinical Supervision and Mentorship in Nursing*. 2nd ed. Stanley Thornes (Publishers) Ltd., Cheltenham.

Fowler J (1996) The organisation of clinical supervision within the nursing profession: a review of the literature. *Journal of Advanced Nursing*, 23: 471–478.

Freshwater D (2002) The therapeutic use of self in nursing. In: Freshwater D (ed.) *Therapeutic Nursing*. Sage Publications, London.

Hawkins P and Shohet R (1989) *Supervision in the Helping Professions. An Individual, Group and Organisational Approach*. Open University Press, Milton Keynes.

Heron J (2001) *Helping the Client. A Creative Practical Guide.* 5th ed. Sage, London.

Johns C (1995) The value of reflective practice for nursing. *Journal of Clinical Nursing*, 2: 307–312.

Johns C (2003) Clinical supervision as a model for clinical leadership. *Journal of Nursing Management*, 11(1): 25–34.

Johns C (2004) Becoming a Reflective Practitioner. 2nd ed. Blackwell Publishing, Oxford.

Johns C (2005) *Transforming Nursing Through Reflective Practice.* 2nd ed. Blackwell Publishing, Oxford.

Jones A (2003) Some benefits experienced by hospice nurses from group clinical supervision. *European Journal of Cancer Care*, 12: 224–232.

Kadushin A (1992) *Supervision in Social Work.* 3rd ed. Columbia University Press, New York.

Mallik (1998) The role of nurse educators in the development of reflective practitioners: A selective case study of the Australian and UK experience. *Nurse Education Today*, 18: 52–63.

Ooijen EG van (1996) Evidence based practice through clinical supervision. Unpublished CRNA conference paper, Oxford.

Pateman B (1998) Clinical supervision in district nursing. In: Butterworth T, Faugier J and Burnard P (eds) *Clinical Supervision and Mentorship in Nursing.* 2nd ed. Stanley Thornes (Publishers) Ltd., Cheltenham.

Pearson A (1998) Excellence in care: Future dimensions for effective nursing. *NTResearch* 3.1. p. 25. Emap Publications, London.

Proctor B (1986) On being a trainer: Training and supervision for counselling in action. In: Hawkins P and Shohet R (eds) *Supervison in the Helping Professions.* Oxford University Press, Milton Keynes.

Revans R W (1976) *Action Learning in Hospitals.* McGraw-Hill.

Rolfe G (1998) *Expanding Nursing Knowledge.* Butterworth Heinemann, Oxford.

Sarafino EP (2002) *Health Psychology. Biopsychosocial Interactions.* 4th ed. Wiley & Sons, New York.

Seligman M E P (1975) *Helplessness: On Depression, Development, and Death.* Freeman, San Francisco.

Smith MK (1996) 'The functions of supervision', *The Encyclopedia of Informal Education*, Last update: 28 January 2005. http://www.infed.org/biblio/functions _of_ supervision.htm

Todd E (2002) The role of the internal supervisor. In: Freshwater D (ed.) *Therapeutic Nursing.* Publications, London.

Walsh K, Nicholson J, Keough C, Pridham R, Kramer M and Jeffrey J (2003) Development of a group model of clinical supervision to meet the needs of a community mental health nursing team. *International Journal of Nursing Practice*, Blackwell Science Ltd.

Wilkin P (1998) Clinical supervision and community psychiatric nursing. In: Butterworth T, Faugier J and Burnard P (eds) *Clinical Supervision and*

Mentorship in Nursing. 2nd ed. Stanley Thornes (Publishers) Ltd., Cheltenham.

Woods D (1992) The use of therapeutic self. In: Butterworth T and Faugier J (eds) *Clinical Supervision and Mentorship in Nursing*. Stanley Thornes (Publishers) Ltd., Cheltenham.

Yegdich T (1999) Clinical supervision: some historical and conceptual considerations. *Journal of Advanced Nursing*, 30(5): 1195–1202.

3

Reflective Practice and Clinical Supervision: Two Sides of the Same Coin?

Dawn Freshwater

SYNOPSIS

In this chapter, the assumed and sometimes poorly articulated relationship between clinical supervision and reflective practice is examined in detail. This is done through a considered discussion of the development of both concepts in the context of the diversity of literature available. Specifically, this chapter explores the underpinning beliefs, values and assumptions of reflective practice and clinical supervision with the aim of highlighting the areas of similarity and difference.

Introduction

This chapter examines the relationship between clinical supervision and reflective practice. It is often assumed that reflective practice is at the heart of clinical supervision and is the foundation of what is sometimes termed guided reflection. Indeed several authors note that clinical supervision involves critical reflection by the supervisee and the supervisor and as such provides an environment within which reflective practice can be fostered (Freshwater 2000; Burton, 2000; Rolfe et al., 2001; Johns and Freshwater, 2005).

However, not all nurse writers concur with the view that reflective practice is integral to clinical supervision, perhaps because the two concepts have been developed almost independently and as such have separate, although interrelated evidence bases. Not surprisingly then the discourse around clinical supervision and reflective practice is at times polarized and often confusing. The aim of this chapter is to explore the assumptions, beliefs and values of both reflective practice and clinical supervision, to clarify how each refers and relates to the other.

Reflection, Reflective Practice and Critical Reflection: Defining the Terms

One of the major challenges for any reader/writer interested in reflection and reflective practice (and indeed clinical supervision) is that of defining the terms. In this next section, my intention is not to provide a prescriptive and static definition of the concepts themselves, rather I aim to make available to the reader a number of perspectives on reflection, both historical and contemporary, by way of positioning the subsequent discussion.

Early attempts at defining reflection drew upon the work of philosophers, one of the earliest being posited by John Dewey (1933; p. 84) who defined reflection as the 'active, persistent and careful consideration of any belief or supposed form of knowledge in the light of the grounds that support it and the further conclusions to which it tends'. Since this early viewpoint, many other writers have followed on with their own definitions, these nearly always linking reflection to learning from experience. Over two decades ago Boyd and Fales (1983) for example described reflection as an internal learning process in which an issue of concern is examined. Thus, meaning is created and clarified in terms of self, resulting in a changed conceptual perspective. Boyd and Fales (1983) asserted here that through reflection the individual may come to see the world differently and as a result of new insights can, in turn, come to act differently. The pivotal part of this definition is that it involves a change in the self; in other words it is not just individual behaviour that has changed but also the individual, hinting at the transformational potential of reflective practice (Freshwater, 1998, 2000, 2002).

A slightly different interpretation of reflection was offered by Johns (1995; p. 24) who over a decade ago defined reflection as: 'the practitioner's ability to access, make sense of and learn through work experience, to achieve more desirable, effective and satisfying work'. For Johns the issue of concern was one that Boyd and Fales (1983) alluded to, and comes from the experience of conflict or cognitive dissonance in practice. Interestingly, this was also the thrust of the work of Arygris and Schon (1974) who discussed the notion of action theories, positing that all human actions reflect ideas, models or some kind of theoretical notion of purpose and intention and ways in which these purposes and intentions can be executed (Rolfe et al., 2001; Freshwater, 1998, 1999, 2000). Agyris and Schon (1974) also noted that people often say one thing and do another. Thus, an individual has a personal theory but when it is operationalised, there is sometimes a contradiction. Based on this idea, they developed the concept of espoused theories, (the stated purpose or intention), and theories in use, (the attempt to put stated intentions or purpose into action). Hence, espoused theories are those to which individuals claim allegiance: theories in use are those theories that are present when action is executed. Human action therefore is never atheoretical or accidental, even if the theory involved in the action is implicit or tacit. Thus it could be argued that reflection is a way of redeeming theories in use which may be tacit and that practice, in this sense, is theory generating (Greenwood, 1998; Freshwater and Avis, 2004).

Reflection then has been, and continues to be, viewed as a significant learning tool with Donald Schon (1983) doing much to expose the role of reflection in professional education. Describing the limitations of knowledge derived from technical rationality for practice, Schon (1983; p. 13) commented that 'the application of research based knowledge to the solution of instrumental choice that dominates the epistemology of professional practice'. Schon also argued that practitioners have difficulty in utilizing this type of knowledge as it is generated in situations that are context free, thereby ignoring the context of the actual practice situation, drawing attention to the fact that practitioners do not as a rule make decisions based on technical rationality, but on experience. Reflective practice has been developed in nursing as a method of accessing and building upon that experiential (and other types of) knowledge.

Schon identified two main aspects of reflective practice, these being reflection on action and in action. Nurses and allied health professionals have adopted, adapted, criticised and further developed Schon's thesis and in particular the concepts of reflection in and on action (Rolfe, 1998; Burton, 2000; Freshwater and Rolfe, 2001; Clouder and Sellars, 2004; Lahteenmaki, 2005). Reflection on action is a retrospective process and as such is the thinking that occurs after an incident with the aim of making sense and using process outcomes to influence future practice. Reflection in action relates to the intuitive art of thinking on one's feet. As mentioned many writers have adopted and developed some of Schon's earlier ideas linking them to reflexivity, reflection before action and the theory practice gap; however, his work has also been subject to some heavy criticism since its publication, mainly with regard to the concept of reflection in action, which it has been suggested, needs further clarification (Day, 1993; Eraut, 1995). Eraut, for example, made a comprehensive critique of Schon's work, arguing that some of his work was unclear. While Eraut might be justified in pointing out the lack of clarity (and perhaps reflection) in Schon's early works, it should of course be noted that these are Eraut's own reflections, which are also open to further refinement and clarification. Further, from the perspective of a reflective practitioner, all work is work in progress!

In the nursing literature, Greenwood (1998) criticised Schon's (1983) model of reflection, arguing that it does not recognise reflection before action; this it would seem is a valid point and one that had been made previously by Reed and Proctor (1993), who wrote about the importance of thinking through a particular situation in advance. Burton (2000; p. 325) wrote that this type of reflection before action is 'an essential precursor to introducing clinical supervision', clearly linking the two concepts. However, it should be noted that this particular view represents a longitudinal view of reflection, based within a linear timeframe, drawing upon Western logic and as such needs to be viewed within that context.

Taylor, who's writing centered on reflection in nursing practice defined reflection as 'the throwing back of thoughts and memories, in cognitive acts such as thinking, contemplation, meditation and any other form of attentive consideration, in order to make sense of them, and to make contextually appropriate changes if they are required' (2000; p. 3). This definition, similar to many others, is permissive in that it allows for a wide variety of thinking and types of knowing as the basis for reflection, suggesting that reflective thinking is both a rational and an intuitive process, which potentiates change. Writing of the technical, practical and emancipatory reflection for holistic practice Taylor described emancipatory reflective practice for overcoming complexities and constraints in holistic health care (Taylor, 2003); provided guidance in technical reflection for improving nursing procedures (Taylor, 2002); and on becoming a reflective nurse or midwife, using complementary therapies while practising holistically (Taylor, 2000).

More recently, Freshwater (2002) has linked the practice of reflection to the essential nursing skill of developing self-awareness. Referring to the therapeutic relationship she comments that reflection helps the practitioner to reform their identity through being in relation with themselves, the patients and others in contrast to having an identity that is formed purely by their surroundings.

According to many theorists reflection has differing levels of depth as well as processes. These levels of reflectivity were discussed in detail by Mezirow (1981, 1990) and although these works are fairly dated in academic terms, they are still viewed as central to the understanding of critical and reflective thinking in both education and health sciences. The levels of reflectivity fall into two broad categories, consciousness and critical consciousness (See Figure 3.1).

Mezirow (1981) suggested the idea of a continuum from consciousness to critical consciousness and eventually towards perspective transformation. There are many examples of nurse educationalists and theorists who have adopted Mezirow's (1981) work in their own explorations of reflectivity. Paget (2001) for instance in his study of practitioners' views of reflective practice impact upon clinical outcomes, identified degrees of perspective transformation across a number of practitioners. Freshwater's (2000) research with student nurses also utilised Mezirow's continuum, linking perspective transformation with transformatory learning through clinical supervision.

One of the consequences of having a range of definitions of reflection is that where reflective practice is concerned a variety of different frameworks have been generated. Such frameworks provide a useful starting point, as the process of constructing an experience

Consciousness	Critical Consciousness
Affective reflectivity	Conceptual reflectivity
Discriminant reflectivity	Psychic reflectivity
Judgmental reflectivity	Theoretical reflectivity

Figure 3.1   Mezirow's (1981) levels of reflectivity.

becomes so taken for granted that we only become aware that it is a process when it is broken down. However, the availability of many reflective frameworks has, it seems, also added to the confusion and lack of clarity surrounding the concept of reflection itself.

Greenwood (1998) explored this idea in depth, presenting two types of framework existing in relation to the process of reflection, these being single and double loop learning. Generating the concept of single and double loop learning from the work of Arygris and Schon (1974) she noted that the reflective practitioner may respond to a reflection on a situation in two ways (although I would argue that this should read *at least* two ways). First, the practitioner may search for an alternative means to achieve the same ends, the actions are changed to achieve the same outcomes, this Greenwood terms single loop learning. Second, the practitioner may respond not only by exploring alternative means to achieve the intended outcomes, but also examines the appropriateness of the chosen ends. Thus double loop learning 'involves reflection on values and norms and, by implication, the social structures which were instrumental in their development and which render them meaningful' (Greenwood, 1998; p. 1049).

This could be interpreted to mean that the practitioner is actively engaged in examining themselves and themselves in relation to the other, in this instance the social structure within which they operate. This type of reflection requires a great deal of self-monitoring and discipline, but encourages learner autonomy by facilitating in the learner the ability to check their own development.

Freshwater (2005a) referred to a similar structure when she noted the distinguishing features of reflection, critical reflection and reflexivity. Simply stated she described reflection as a focussed way of thinking about practice, whatever that practice is. Practices are subject to a degree of scrutiny and examination with the aim of achieving a deeper awareness and understanding of that practice. Critical reflection differs in that the practitioner is not only thinking about their current practices, they are also subjecting the way they are thinking about practice to a degree of interrogation. In other words, the practitioner is thinking about how they are thinking, while simultaneously thinking about their practice. Our ways of thinking have been heavily socialised not only by professional training and academic learning, but also by political, ethical, historical and cultural traditions. As such our thinking is both constructed by our contextual position, and as we exist in that contextual position, we also contribute to constructing it. Having an awareness of this meta-level of contextual influence on both our thinking and our practices and bringing it to bear through reflective processes is termed reflexivity. (Reflexivity is both a method of collecting data about practice and a research method in its own right.) In this sense Freshwater and Rolfe (2001) differentiated reflexivity as a turning back on itself and a type of meta-reflection, emphasising its critical nature of unsettling previously held assumptions to gain new awareness. This, they argued is a fundamental purpose of clinical supervision.

On reading the literature it would be easy to slip into devising a hierarchy of reflection, as Greenwood (1998) does, considering double loop learning to be superior to single loop learning and indeed this could also be an interpretation of Freshwater's (2005a) work. However, this is not useful as it argues for a gap reminiscent of the theory–practice gap in nursing. And while it might seem obvious to point it out, deep learning can only be made known by coming to the surface. Similarly reflection and critical reflection are precursors to reflexivity and as such are interdependent. It would seem preferable to advocate an approach to reflection that provides a structure within which structures can be deconstructed. In other words, a reflective framework needs to be used flexibly and dynamically. Indeed all work surrounding reflection and its development needs to be relative and evolutionary, paralleling the true nature of reflection (and indeed clinical practice) itself. It could be argued that one such structure is that of clinical supervision, that is to say that clinical supervision could be simply described as a flexible and dynamic structure within which to continuously deconstruct and reconstruct clinical practice. I will come back to this at a later point in the chapter.

While outlining the term(s) itself may have caused a few conceptual headaches, it would seem from the literature that it is easier to describe the processes of reflection and it is to this that I will now turn my attention. However, before moving on there is one further comment to be made regarding the arrival at a single definition of reflection. Taking up the point made by Atkins and Murphy (1993), that if authors do not share a common definition of reflection then it is difficult to make comparisons across studies, which in turn makes it difficult to assess the value of reflection in influencing patient outcomes. This seems to miss the point that reflection is an individual process of learning that reflects individual experience and meaning. It is, by its very nature, localised, and there will therefore be some differences in how it is understood and processed and at the same time there will be some shared commonalties which can be transferred across discipline, settings and practices.

Reflective Practice and the Development of Expertise

The Process of Reflection

What the literature regarding reflection does have in common is that the complex *process* of reflection is discussed. It is the process of reflection that can be best captured and facilitated in the process of clinical supervision. Most authors have identified stages or levels of reflection, Mezirow (1981). Levels of reflectivity have been indicated previously, Schon (1983) identified three levels of reflection, these being reflection, criticism and action; others have also been posited. Atkins and Murphy (1993), in their assessment of the literature, discovered that there were three key stages in the reflective process that were shared by most authors. Figure 3.2 attempts to synthesise some of these. Several authors devised reflective cycles to illustrate the integral and circular nature of the reflective process (Kolb, 1984). It is

First Stage	**Awareness of uncomfortable feelings and thoughts** – experience of surprise – inner discomfort – affective, discriminant, judgmental reflectivity
Second Stage	**Critical analysis of the situation** – reflection and criticism – openness to new information and perspectives; resolution – conceptual, psychic and theoretical reflectivity – association, integration, validation and appropriation
Third Stage	**Development of new perspective** – establishing continuity of self with past, present and future; deciding whether and how to take action – perspective transformation – cognitive, affective and behavioural changes – action

Figure 3.2   The processes of reflection.

this reflection as praxis that integrates reflection before action into the reflective process in a non-linear manner involving ongoing development of the practitioner.

Reflection-in-action it is argued also involves three distinct, but inextricable intertwined processes, McCleod (1996) identified these as:

- Noticing - a conscious awareness that can be enhanced.
- Reflection - past experiences and understanding, plus the particulars of the present context with the practitioner deeply immersed in the unfolding situation. (Although McCleod did not refer to reflection-in-action her understanding is described as reflexive, flexible and responsive).
- Action/Intervening - selecting from a range of options.

The smooth flowing, tightly bound nature of these components means that while reflection-in-action can be developed, analysis is rarely complete and reflection on action is generally required for deeper understanding with the potential for perspective transformation (Taylor et al., 2005). During this dynamic process the practitioner creates a space within which to view their espoused theories, beliefs and values alongside their theories in action with the intent of uncovering contradictions. As the practitioner becomes more aware of their own 'guiding fictions' so the possibility of choice, intentionality and deliberative nursing practice become more of a reality. McLeod (1996; p. 136) explicated this move to intentional practice succinctly saying that 'The possibility of choice arises from reflexivity, since the person does not respond automatically to events but acts intentionally based on awareness of alternatives'.

As a process then reflective practice is multidimensional and seeks to problematise a broad range of professional situations encountered by the practitioner so that they can become potential learning situations (Boyd and Fales, 1983; Schon, 1983; Greenwood, 1998; Johns and Freshwater, 1998; Burton, 2000; Clouder and Sellars, 2004; Lahteenmaki, 2005). Thus reflection enables a continuation of learning and development in which the practitioner grows in and through their practice (Todd and Freshwater, 1999; Randle, 2002). Or as Burton (2000; p. 326) writes, 'Reflection is a means of formalizing informal learning and development through practice and can be used in the development of the professional portfolio'. Importantly, the practitioner develops an intentionality in regard to practice that has the potential to impact patient care and to refine and define good practice. In this sense, reflective practice should be and is increasingly located as central to practice development, advanced nursing practice and expert practice (Benner, 1984; Glaze, 1998; Johns, 1998; Rolfe, 1998; Burton, 2000; Rolfe et al., 2001; Johns and Freshwater, 2005). While the interpretation of what constitutes an expert practitioner continues to be expanded and refined, what is clear is that the practitioner with 'conscious expertise' is one that has a willingness to reflect, is willing to learn from experience, is open minded and does not function in isolation (Dewey, 1933). Interestingly, all that has been said so far about reflective practice has also been reported concerning clinical supervision, almost word for word in some instances. And so the reader might ask, rightly so, what is the difference between the two? I hope that by the end of this chapter it will become obvious that there are fewer differences than there are similarities.

It is largely agreed that practice development nurses, clinical nurse specialists and nurse consultants act as experts, providing guidance on the development and implementation of best practice, supporting research, innovation and change, and encouraging professional development. Few would disagree that practice development requires that practitioners have opportunities to critically appraise their work (and that of others) to ensure that practice is evidence based. To this end many of the advanced practitioners referred to above act as clinical supervisors, facilitating a parallel process to practice development and providing an opportunity for doing the same (see Figure 3.3).

Reflective practice can be seen as a companion and precursor to practice development in many ways. Not only does it help to assess if practice behaviour is congruent with espoused values and beliefs, it also assists in the development of autonomy through self-monitoring (Freshwater, 1998) and accountability through shared learning such as in clinical supervision. Mezirow (1991) considered reflection vital for the building of competence; referring to the process of critical reflection he contends that questioning the validity of previous learning can lead to a regeneration of knowledge, which in turn produces new or changed meanings. Burton (2000) took this idea one step further and explicitly linked clinical supervision, reflective practice and the development of competence (referring to Benner's framework...ref.. and that of Blake and Blanchard...ref..). In addition it can prevent complacency in everyday practice, which it has been argued, can lead to routinised practice (Walsh and Ford, 1989). As

Level of Reflection	Methods of Reflection	Stages of Development
Descriptive	Reflective diaries, reporting incidents Reflection on action	Practice becomes Conscious
Dialogic	Discourse with peers in various arenas including clinical supervision	Practice becomes Deliberative
Critical	Able to provide reasoning for actions by engaging in critical conversation with Practice/Self/Others	Transformation of Practice/practice Development/innovation

Figure 3.3 Model of reflection for practice development (Freshwater, 1998).

already mentioned effective reflection on practice can lead to more conscious, deliberative and intentional interventions. Furthermore, reflection on beliefs, values and norms offers the opportunity to examine, articulate and generate local philosophies and theories of care, as well as assessing the contribution that individuals make to health care delivery at a national level. The generation and assessment of informal theory is something that is inherent in both the process of reflection and in the development of practice.

Models of reflective practice are numerous, just as there is an abundance of models for framing clinical supervision. Models of reflection not only provide a way of redeeming theories in use, emphasising the importance of theorising about knowledge grounded in practice, they also represent a dialectic between knowing and doing, regarding practice as a base for knowledge generation (Benner, 1984; Lumby, 1998). Models also enable the practitioner to grasp the purpose of reflective practice, which are sometimes only implied within the specified framework.

Argyris and Schön (1974) viewed the purpose of reflective practice as the creation of a world that more faithfully reflects the values and beliefs of people in it, through the construction or revision of peoples' action theories (Greenwood, 1998). Greenwood (1998; p. 2) provided a comprehensive summary of the purposes of reflection based on a synthesis of other writer's views. Adapted and updated this is as follows:

- develop individual theories of nursing, to influence practice and generate nursing knowledge (Emden, 1991; Reid, 1993);
- advance theory at a conceptual level to lead to changes at professional, social and political levels (Emden, 1991; Smyth, 1992, 1993);
- facilitate integration of theory and practice (McCougherty, 1991; Wong et al., 1995; Landeen et al., 1995);
- allow the correction of distortions and errors in beliefs related to discrete activities, and the values and norms that underpin them (Mezirow, 1990);
- encourage a holistic, individualised and flexible approach to care (Freshwater, 2002; Parker, 2002);
- allow the identification, description and resolution of practical problems through deliberative rationalisation (Powell, 1989);
- enhance self-esteem through learning (Johns, 1994, 1995; Freshwater, 2000; Randle, 2002);
- heighten the visibility of the therapeutic work of nurses (Johns, 1994, 1995; Freshwater, 2002);
- enable the monitoring of increasing effectiveness over time (Johns, 1995; Landeen et al., 1995);
- enable nurses to explore and come to understand the nature and boundaries of their own role and that of other health professionals (Johns, 1994, 1995; Freshwater, 2002);
- lead to an understanding of the condition under which practitioners practise and, in particular, the barriers that limit the practitioners' therapeutic value (Emden, 1991; Johns, 1994, 1995);
- lead to an acceptance of professional responsibility (Johns, 1994, 1995);
- allow a shift in the social control of work. Less direct, overt surveillance over work and much more indirect forms of control through, for example teamwork, partnerships, collaboration, etc. (Smyth, 1992, 1993; Gilbert, 2001; Clouder and Sellars, 2004);
- provide the opportunity to shift the power to determine what counts as knowledge from an elite, distant from the workplace, to practitioners in the workplace (Smyth, 1992, 1993; Freshwater and Rolfe, 2004);
- allow the generation of a knowledge base that is more comprehensive because it is directly tuned into what practitioners know about practice (Smyth, 1992, 1993); and

- provide the opportunity for a rapid and progressive refocusing of work activity (Smyth, 1992, 1993).

More recent work by Taylor et al. (2005) identified several tangential purposes of reflective practice, including the creation of spiritual awareness through reflection to address spiritual needs for self and assisting the patient; the development of emotional literacy and emotional intelligence (self-discovery, self-awareness, self-management, motivation, and empathy) for self-transformation (Freshwater, 2004); and the expansion of leadership capacity as a transformative change agent (Sherwood and Freshwater, 2005).

In addition, Taylor et al. (2005) asserted that:

> The goal of reflective practice is always in a positive direction, for the growth and discovery of self and one's knowledge, progressing the ability to integrate into one's deepening and expanded practice. In other words, the list of purposes grows as each new venture into reflective practice provides evidence of the usefulness of it, for a wide range of uses in every field of nursing.

There are numerous strategies identified in the literature to promote the development of reflection, critical reflection and reflexivity. These include journaling, role play, critical incident technique among many others (See Taylor et al., 2005). One such strategy is that of clinical supervision, and it is to this that the remainder of this chapter is dedicated.

Facilitating Reflective Practice through Clinical Supervision

It has been noted that there are a variety of ways in which the skills of critical reflection can be acquired, and that clinical supervision is one such way (Taylor et al., 2005; Johns and Freshwater, 2005). While clinical supervision is a fairly new concept in nursing, it has a long tradition in such disciplines as counseling, psychotherapy, social work and midwifery. Rolfe et al. (2001) noted that initial interest in supervision in the United Kingdom developed as a direct result of two publications, these being the Vision for the Future (DoH, 1993) and the position paper on clinical supervision commissioned by the Department of Health (Faugier and Butterworth, 1994). The UKCC

(1996) responded to these publications by highlighting the importance of adequate standards of supervision.

An area that continues to be debated is that of the facilitation of reflective practice; just as practice cannot be changed in isolation, it is argued that practitioners struggle to objectify their own beliefs, values and actions without the benefit of another perspective. Burton (2000) argued that reflection needs to be guided, referring to the earlier works of Johns (1996) and Cox et al. (1991); she advocated support from a skilled supervisor. Clinical supervision, the focus of this book, is linked explicitly with practice development (UKCC, 1996), and appears to some extent to have been reified as the ideal forum within which to foster reflective practice. Definitions of clinical supervision abound and can be found throughout this and many other books, thus I will not deal with this aspect of supervision in any detail here. However, I will repeat my earlier statement regarding the role of clinical supervision and reflective practice by way of establishing my own particular preference. This was that clinical supervision could be simply described as a flexible and dynamic structure within which to continuously deconstruct and reconstruct clinical practice. At this stage I wish to add that fundamental to this process of deconstruction and reconstruction are the skills of reflection, critical reflection and reflexivity. In other words, clinical supervision and reflective practice are interdependent and inextricably linked through the process of reflection.

While it would not be true to say that all the literature around clinical supervision emphasise the skills of reflection it is fair to say that the two concepts are often described concurrently. Many models of clinical supervision are presented, nearly all of which include an element of reflection and reflection on practice (Hawkins and Shohet, 1989; Holloway, 1995; Bond and Holland, 1998); others suggest reflection is itself a model for supervision (Todd and Freshwater, 1999; Johns, 2000; Van Ooijen, 2000; Rolfe et al., 2001; Freshwater and Johns, 2005). In addition, some of the most widely used definitions of clinical supervision make reflective practice central to the aims of supervision. In 1994 Kohner, for example, identified the main purpose of clinical supervision as that of facilitating reflective practice within a patient-centred focus, a view that is supported by several authors who propose that clinical supervision offers an ideal setting for the guidance of reflective practice.

Whereas some nursing commentators have questioned whether or not reflective practice needs to be an integral part of clinical supervision (Fowler and Chevannes, 1998), others have examined the relationship in detail. Todd and Freshwater (1999; p. 1383), for example, examined the 'parallels and processes of a model of reflection in an individual clinical supervision session, and the use of guided discovery'. The authors advocate reflective practice as a model for clinical supervision 'because it provides safe space that facilitates a collaborative and empowering relationship which enables the practitioner to experience a journey of discovery in examining his/her everyday practice' (Todd and Freshwater, 1999; p. 1388). Heath and Freshwater (2000; p. 1298) used John's (1996) 'intent-emphasis axis to explore how a technical interest, misunderstanding of expert practice, and confusion of self awareness with counselling, can detract from the supervisory process'. They examined the nature of clinical supervision and reflective practice and how the two can combine effectively, especially when supervisors are reflective about their roles, and the clinical supervision experience is a guided reflection that enables deeper insights for the supervisee and supervisor.

On a slightly different track, Gilbert (2001; p. 199) focused on the 'meticulous rituals of the confessional' and the potential for reflective practice and clinical supervision to act as 'modes of surveillance disciplining the action of professionals'. Using Foucault's (1982) concept of governmentality, Gilbert argued that, like governments, health settings act as 'forms of moral regulation' in which professionals exercise power through 'the complex web of discourses and social practices that characterize their work' (Gilbert, 2001; p. 199). In critiquing the discourses of empowerment that underlie the emancipatory intent of reflective practice and clinical supervision, he identified the tendency of empowerment discourses to assume 'the existence of a damaged subject-traditional and rule bound (who) requires remedial work ... to achieve forms of subjectivity consistent with modern forms of rule' (Gilbert, 2001; p. 205).

Clouder and Sellars (2004; p. 262), writing from the perspective of physiotherapists, used research conducted with undergraduate occupational therapy and physiotherapist students to 'contribute to the debate about the functions of clinical supervision and reflective practice in nursing and other health care professions'. The authors responded to Gilbert's (2001) criticism of the sterility of debates about reflection and clinical supervision, and the potential for moral regulation and surveillance. They concluded that although both strategies make individuals more visible within the gaze of the workplace, that Gilbert 'overlooked the possibility of resistance and the scope for personal agency within systems of surveillance that create tensions between personal and professional accountability'.

Freshwater (2005b) to some extent agreed with Gilbert, in that she stated: 'it could be posited that reflection guided through clinical supervision monitors the level of deviance from protocols, codes of conduct and policies, this through a confessional practice'. However, turning Foucault's theory back on itself, she, like Cloud and Sellars (2004) pointed toward the scope for subversion and agency within the supervisory arrangement itself, providing examples of studies conducted in secure environments (Freshwater et al., 2001, 2002; Freshwater, 2005).

It could be argued that this view is heavily dependant upon the orientation of the facilitator. Lahteenmaki (2005) observed that the supervision that students receive is closely related to their supervisor's view of the goals of learning; other writers concur with this view (see, for example, Van Ooijen). As an illustration of this, in the apprentice–master approach to learning, which relies heavily on the technical instrumental philosophy of education, the supervisee/practitioner is viewed as a passive recipient of knowledge. By way of contrast, reflective and critical approaches to learning, which emphasise the role of the supervisee/practitioner in analysing and understanding their own practices, concentrate on eliciting the supervisee's espoused theories and values. To this end, reflective practice is an integral part of clinical supervision that focuses on facilitating learning through empowerment and emancipation (Freshwater, 2000; Taylor, 2002, 2004). Naturally, some individuals respond better to the apprentice–master approach to learning, finding reflection threatening and challenging, most often because it forces them to reflect on and develop an inner authority through the constant testing out of personal and relational hypotheses. But to argue for a supervision practice that either includes or dismisses reflective practice serves only to dichotomise the two concepts, and does little to acknowledge the interdependence of the two. Most experienced facilitators of learning would point out that the real skill of supervision is in integrating facilitative and directive skills to enable an optimal learning environment to suit the individual needs of the practitioner/learner.

Reflection, Research and Evidence-based Practice

Criticisms of reflective practice mainly centre on its failure to demonstrate its usefulness through research studies. Day (1993), for example, pointed out that how reflection changes practice is unknown. This criticism stemmed from the argument that the studies that have been carried out related only to the process of reflection and the practitioner's experience (Hargreaves, 1997). These criticisms are rebuked in the literature as missing the point that the value of reflection is inherent in the experience of the process. As Heath (1998; p. 291) argued 'Reflective practice focuses on practice 'as it is' and aims to enhance practice from that starting point... .' The positivist voice is criticised as ignoring the focus of reflective practice as a starting point in favour of a defining point (Heath, 1998).

There is, however, some evidence, albeit minimal, that reflective practice has links with client outcomes. Powell (1989) attempted to access tacit knowledge, often described as defying explanation, using reflection. Powell's (1989) study used Mezirow's levels of reflectivity as signposts to monitor the depth of reflection undertaken by a group of practitioners. Although a small sample was used in this local study, it provides a useful benchmark for development to explore how levels of reflection may enhance practice outcomes. Other studies build upon Powell's (1989) earlier work and indicate that increased depth of reflectivity equates with improved patient care (Freshwater, 1998). Research studies that have examined the link between reflection and client care include Gray and Forsstrom (1991), McCaugherty (1991), Crandall and Getchell-Reiter (1993), Hodgston (1995) and Johns (1998a).

Though sceptics in the literature accept that reflection offers valuable insight into interactions surrounding client care (Tolley, 1995), the main area of contention continues to be about the relatively small gains that are accumulated over time by individual practitioners. It would appear that to be of value, benefits must be large and rapid with measurable outcomes (Heath, 1998). Unfortunately, the experiential knowledge embedded in everyday practice, and embodied in the subsequent practice narratives, is still judged using scientific measures and is caught in a competitive dialogue with empirical knowledge. This does little to progress the development of reflective strategies as Lumby (1998; p. 93) pointed out:

> Reflection as a research tool or method continues to be perceived as questionable as far as issues of validity, reliability and generalization are concerned, often forcing nurses to abandon such strategies or to manipulate them in a way which ensures loss of integrity.

Resulting in evidence-based practice, reflection and practice development become dichotomised and reminiscent of the theory–practice gap.

Newell (1994), it seems, was closer to the mark when he argued, with some vehemence, that reflection needs to be defined in a way that allows its efficacy on nurses and client care to be tested. This is not only a valid point but allows for individual definitions of reflection to be operationalised in the pursuit of evidence-based practice. It is my argument in this chapter that clinical supervision is one way of defining reflective practice (and critical reflection) that allows and provides opportunities for efficacy and impact studies, should nursing and allied health professionals be willing to accept the assertion that reflection and clinical supervision are two sides of the same coin.

Conclusion

In conclusion then, reflection offers a way of accessing deeply embedded personal knowledge. Schon (1983) purported that thinking, via reflection, adds theory to the action while it is occurring, making theory and practice inseparable. Contemporary literature juxtaposes the skills of reflection, the reflective cycle and learning from experience with the skills of clinical supervision.

It could be argued that the event of clinical supervision, and the subsequent literature, has done much to add to the development and understanding of the application of reflective practice in nursing (and vice versa). It has provided clear frameworks for the structure and implementation of the abstract concept of clinical supervision. There does however remain some unanswered questions, both in relation to reflective practice and clinical supervision. Namely, what difference does it make? The answer to this and other associated questions are constantly being evaluated, and while tentative answers are now beginning to emerge in the nursing literature, the gap in this area continues to exist.

To facilitate reflective practice supervisors must allocate time for students to discuss fully a clinical situation, to identify and challenge assumptions, beliefs, values, and ideologies that underlie nursing practice. Supervisors must create a balance between listening, supporting and confronting, to facilitate the reasoning process and create grounded conceptual frameworks in nursing practice (Rolfe et al., 2001; Freshwater, 2002).

It would seem then that the literature concerning reflective practice and clinical supervision, quite aptly, is in process, is deliberative and like clinical practice is continuously evolving. While the definitions of reflection are flexible and dynamic, mirroring the process of learning from experience, there is some agreement on what the process of reflection involves. Namely, an awareness of uncomfortable feelings and thoughts, followed by a critical analysis of feelings and knowledge leading to the development of a new perspective.

The infusion of reflective practice in healthcare demands that awareness and evaluation of self, experience and others is not only a recommended skill but also a requisite of healthcare education, an issue that the literature on experiential learning refers to. Further, in as much as nursing appears to have embraced the concept of reflection, in theory, the literature challenges the practitioner (researcher) to further develop methods of assessing the value of reflective practice in practice. Perhaps clinical supervision provides a forum within which this evaluation can take place. Hence the prevailing question (and therein the gap in the literature) remains: How does clinical supervision make a difference?

References

Argyris C and Schön DA (1974) *Theory in Practice: Increasing Professional Effectiveness*. Jossey Bass: Washington, DC.

Atkins S and Murphy K (1993) Reflection: A review of the literature. *Journal of Advanced Nursing*, 18: 1188–1192.

Benner P (1984) *From Novice to Expert: Uncovering the Knowledge Embedded in Clinical Practice*. Addison-Wesley, California.

Bond M and Holland S (1998) *Skills of Clinical Supervision for Nurses*. Open University Press: Milton Keynes.

Boyd EM and Fales AW (1983). Reflective learning: key to learning from experience. *Journal of Humanistic Psychology*, 23(2): 99–117.

Burton A (2000) Reflection: nursing's practice and education panacea? *Journal of Advanced Nursing*, 31(5): 1009–1017.

Butterworth T (1998) Clinical supervision as an emerging idea in nursing. In: Butterworth T, Faugier J and Burnard P (eds) *Clinical Supervision and Mentorship in Nursing*. Stanley Thornes, Cheltenham, pp. 1–18.

Clouder L and Sellars J (2004) Reflective practice and clinical supervision: an interprofessional perspective. *Journal of Advanced Nursing*, 46(3): 262–269.

Crandall B and Getchell-Reiter IC (1993) Critical decision method: in a technique for eliciting concrete assessment indicators from the intuitions of NICU nurses. *Advances in Nursing Science*, 16(1): 42–51.

Day C (1993) Research and the continuing professional development of teachers. An inaugural lecture. University of Nottingham: School of Education.

Department of Health (1999) Making a difference, Strengthening the Nursing, Midwifery and Health Visitors' contribution to Health Care. The Stationary Office, London.

Department of Health (1993) A Vision for the Future: The Nursing, Midwifery and Health Visiting Contribution to Health and Health Care. HMSO, London.

Dewey J (1933) *How We Think: A Restatement of the Relation of Reflective Thinking to the Education Process*. Heath, Boston.

Durahee T (1997) Reflective practice: Decoding ethical knowledge. *Nursing Ethics*, 4 (3): 211–217.

Emden C (1991) Becoming a reflective practitioner. In: Gray G and Pratt R (eds) *Towards a Discipline of Nursing*. Churchill Livingstone, Melbourne, pp. 335–354.

Eraut M (1995) Schon shock: A case for reframing reflection-in-action? *Teachers and Teaching*, 1: 9–21.

Faugier J and Butterworth T (1994) *Clinical Supervision: A Position Paper*. Manchester University, Manchester.

Fowler J and Chevannes M (1998) Evaluating the efficacy of reflective practice within the context of clinical supervision. *Journal of Advanced Nursing*, 27: 379–382.

Freshwater D (1998a) The Philosophers Stone. In: Johns C and Freshwater D (eds) *Transforming Nursing Through Reflective Practice*. Blackwell Science, Oxford, Ch. 9.

Freshwater D (1998b) From acorn to oak tree: a neoplatonic perspective of reflection and caring. *Australian Journal of Holistic Nursing*, 5(2): 14–19.

Freshwater D (1999) Communicating with self through caring: the student nurse's experience of reflective practice. *International Journal of Human Caring*, 3(3): 28–33.

Freshwater D (2000) Transformatory Learning in Nurse Education. PhD thesis: University of Nottingham.

Freshwater D (Ed.) (2002). *Therapeutic Nursing: Improving Patient Care Through Reflection*. Sage, London.

Freshwater D (2004) Reflection: A tool for developing clinical leadership. *Reflections on Nursing Leadership*. 2nd Quarter, 20–26.

Freshwater D (2005a) Reflexive Pragmatism, The Natural Harmonic of Caring. 27th International Association for Human Caring, Keynote Address. Lake Tahoe June.

Freshwater D (2005b) Clinical supervision in the context of custodial care. In: Johns C and Freshwater D (eds) *Transforming Nursing Through Reflective Practice*. Blackwell Publishing, Oxford, Ch. 5.

Freshwater D and Avis M (2004) Analysing interpretation and reinterpreting analysis. *Nursing Philosophy.*

Freshwater D and Rolfe G (2001) Critical reflexivity: a politically and ethically engaged method for nursing. *NT Research*, 6(1): 526–537.

Freshwater D and Rolfe G (2004). *Deconstructing Evidence Based Practice.* Taylor and Francis, London.

Freshwater D, Walsh L and Storey L (2001) Developing leadership through clinical supervision in prison healthcare. *Nursing Management*, 8(8): 10.

Freshwater D, Walsh L and Storey L (2002) Developing leadership through clinical supervision in prison healthcare. *Nursing Management*, 2.

Gilbert T (2001) Reflective practice and supervision: meticulous rituals of the confessional. *Journal of Advanced Nursing*, 36(2): 199–205.

Glaze J (1998) Reflection and Expert Nursing Knowledge. In: Johns C and Freshwater D (1998) *Transforming nursing through reflective practice*. Blackwell Science: Oxford, Ch. 12.

Gray J and Forsstom S (1991) Generating theory from practice: the reflective technique. In: Gray G and Pratt R (eds) Towards a discipline of nursing. Chruchill Livingstone: London.

Greenwood J (1993b) Reflective practice: a critique of the work of Argyris and Schön. *Journal of Advanced Nursing*, 18: 1183–1187.

Greenwood J (1998) The role of reflection in single and double loop learning. *Journal of Advanced Nursing Practice*, 27(5): 1048–1053.

Hargreaves J (1997) Using patients: exploring the ethical dimensions of reflective practice in nurse education. *Journal of Advanced Nursing*, 25(2): 223–228.

Hawkins P and Shohet R (1989) *Supervision in the helping professions*. Open University Press: Buckingham.

Heath H (1998) Paradigm, dialogues and dogma: finding a place for research, nursing models and reflective practice. *Journal of Advanced Nursing*, 28(2): 288–294.

Heath H and Freshwater D (2000) Clinical supervision as an emancipatory process: avoiding inappropriate intent. *Journal of Advanced Nursing*, 32(5): 1298–1306.

Hodgston R (1995) Evaluating quality nursing care through peer review and reflection: the findings of a qualitative study. *International Journal of Nursing Studies*, 12(2): 162–172.

Holloway E (1995) *Clinical Supervision: A systems approach.* Sage: London.

Jarvis P (1992) Reflective practice in nursing. *Nursing Education Today*, 12: 174–181.

Johns C (1996) Visualizing and realizing caring in practice through guided reflection. *Journal of Advanced Nursing*, 24: 1135–1143.

Johns C (1994) Nuances of reflection. *Journal of Clinical Nursing*, 3: 71–75.

Johns C and Freshwater D (1998) *Transforming Nursing Through Reflective Practice*. Blackwell Science, Oxford.

Johns C and Freshwater D (2005) *Transforming Nursing Through Reflective Practice*. 2nd Ed. Blackwell Publishing, Oxford.

Johns C (1995) Framing learning through reflection within Carper's fundamental ways of knowing in nursing. *Journal of Advanced Nursing*, 22: 226–234.

Johns, C. (1998) Opening the Doors of perception. In: Johns C and Freshwater D (1998) (eds) *Transforming Nursing through reflective practice*. Blackwell Science: Oxford, Ch 1.

Johns C (2004) Becoming a transformational leader through reflection. *Reflections on Nursing Leadership*, 2nd Quarter 24–26.

Johns PR (2000) *Becoming A Reflective Practitioner*. Blackwell Science, London.

Kolb D (1984) *Experiential Learning as the Science of Learning and Development*. Englewood Cliffs, Prentice Hall, New York.

Lahteenmaki M-L (2005) Reflectivity in supervised practice: conventional and transformative approaches to physiotherapy. *Learning in Health and Social Care*, 4 (1): 18–28.

Landeen J, Byrne D and Brown B (1995) Exploring the lived experiences of psychiatric nursing students through self-reflective journals. *Journal of Advanced Nursing*, 21(5): 878–885.

Lumby J (1998) Transforming nursing through reflective practice. In Johns C and Freshwater D (eds) *Transforming nursing through reflective practice*. Blackwell Science: Oxford, Ch. 8.

McCaugherty, D. (1991) The use of a teaching model to promote reflection and the experiential integration of theory and practice in first year student nurses: an action research study. *Journal of Advanced Nursing*, 16: 534–543.

McCormack B (1995) The development of clinical leadership through supported reflective practice. *Journal of Clinical Nursing*, 4(3): 161–168.

McCougherty D (1991) The theory-practice gap in nurse education: its causes and possible solutions. Findings from an action research study. *Journal of Advanced Nursing*, 16: 1055–1061.

Mezirow J (1991) *Transformative Dimensions of Adult Learning*. Jossey Bass, Oxford.

Mezirow J (1990) How critical reflection triggers transformative learning. In: Mezirow et al. (eds) *Fostering Critical Reflection in Adulthood*, Jossey Bass, San Francisco, pp. 1–20.

Mezirow J (1981) A critical theory of adult learning and education. *Adult Education*, 32: 3–24.

Newell R (1994) Reflection: art, science or pseudo-science. *Nursing Education Today*, 14: 79-81.

Paget T (2001) Reflective practice and clinical outcomes: practitioners' views on how reflective practice has influenced their clinical practice. *Journal of Clinical Nursing*, 10: 204–214.

Parker M (2002) Aesthetic ways in day to day nursing. In: Freshwater D (ed.) *Therapeutic Nursing*. Sage: London, Ch. 6.

Powell JH (1989) The reflective practitioner in nursing. *Journal of Advanced Nursing*, 14(10): 824-832.

Pryce A (2002) Refracting experience: reflection, postmodernity and transformations. *NT Research*, 7(4):298-311.

Randle J (2002) Transformative Learning: Enabling Therapeutic Nursing. In Freshwater D (ed.) *Therapeutic Nursing*. Sage: London, Ch. 5.

Reed J and Procter S (1993) *Nursing Education: A Reflective Approach*. Edward Arnold, London.

Reid B (1993) But we're doing it already! Exploring a response to the concept of reflective practice in order to improve its facilitation. *Nurse Education Today*, 13: 305-309.

Richardson G and Maltby II (1995) Reflection-on-practice. Enhancing student learning. *Journal of Advanced Nursing*, 22 (2): 235-242.

Rolfe G (1998) *Expanding Nursing Knowledge*. Butterworth Heinnemann: Oxford.

Rolfe G (2003) Is there a place for reflection in the nursing curriculum? A reply to Newell. *Clinical Effectiveness in Nursing*, 7(1): 61.

Rolfe G, Freshwater D and Jasper M (2001) *Critical Reflection for Nurses and the Caring Professions: A Users Guide*. Palgrave, Basingstoke.

Schön DA (1983) *The Reflective Practitioner: How Practitioners Think in Action*. Basic Books, New York.

Schön DA (1987) *Educating the Reflective Practitioner*. Jossey-Bass, London.

Schön DA (1991) *The Reflective Practitioner*. 2nd Ed. Jossey Bass, San Francisco.

Sherwood G and Freshwater D (2005) Doctoral education for transformational leadership in a global context. In: Ketefian S and McKenna H (eds) *Doctoral Education in Nursing: International Perspectives*. Routledge, London.

Smith A (1998) Learning about reflection. *Journal of Advanced Nursing*, 28(4): 891-895.

Smyth J (1992) Teachers' work and the politics of reflection. *American Education Research Journal*, 29(2): 267-300.

Smyth J (1993) Reflective Practice in Teacher Education and Other Professions, Key Address to the Fifth National Practicum Conference, Macquarie University, Sydney.

Stickley T and Freshwater D (2002) The art of loving and the therapeutic relationship. *Nursing Inquiry*, 9(4): 250-256.

Street A (1992). *Inside Nursing: A Critical Ethnography of Clinical Nursing*, SUNY, New York.

Stringer ET (1996) *Action Research: a Handbook for Practitioners*. Sage Publications, Thousand Oaks.

Taylor BJ (2000) *Reflective Practice: A Guide for Nurses and Midwives*. UK, Allen and Unwin, Melbourne/Open University Press.

Taylor BJ (2001) Identifying and transforming dysfunctional nurse-nurse relationships through reflective practice and action research. *International Journal of Nursing Practice*, 7(6): 406-413.

Taylor BJ (1997) Big battles for small gains: A cautionary note for teaching reflective processes in midwifery and midwifery. *Midwifery Inquiry*, 4: 19–26.

Taylor B J (2002a) Technical reflection for improving nursing and midwifery procedures using critical thinking in evidence based practice. *Contemporary Nurse*, 13 (2–3): 281–287.

Taylor BJ (2002b) Becoming a reflective nurse or midwife: using complementary therapies while practising holistically. *Complementary Therapies in Nursing and Midwifery*, 8(4): 62–68.

Taylor BJ (2003) Emancipatory reflective practice for overcoming complexities and constraints in holistic health care. *Sacred Space*, 4(2): 40–45.

Taylor BJ (2004) Technical, practical and emancipatory reflection for practising holistically. *Journal of Holistic Nursing*, 22(1): 73–84.

Taylor C (2003) Issues and innovations in nursing education – narrating practice: reflective accounts and the textual construction of reality. *Journal of Advanced Nursing*, 42(3): 244.

Taylor B J, Bulmer B, Hill L, Luxford C, McFarlane J, Stirling K (2002) Exploring idealism in palliative nursing care through reflective practice and action research. *International Journal of Palliative Nursing*, 8(7): 324–330.

Taylor B, Freshwater D, and Sherwood G (2005) Report of the STT Reflective Practice Taskforce.

Teekman B (2000) Exploring reflective thinking in nursing practice. *Journal of Advanced Nursing*, 31(5): 1125–1135.

Todd G and Freshwater D (1999) Reflective practice and guided discovery: clinical supervision. *British Journal of Nursing*, 8(20): 1383–1389.

Tolley K (1995) Theory from practice for practice: is this a reality. *Journal of Advanced Nursing*, 21(1): 184–190.

United Kingdom Central Council (1996) Position statement on clinical supervision for nursing and health visiting, UKCC, London.

United Kingdom Central Council of Nursing Midwifery and Health Visiting (1999) Fitness for practice: The UKCC commission for nursing and midwifery education. UKCC, London.

Van Ooijen E 2000 Clinical Supervision: A Practical Guide. Churchill Livingstone: London.

Walsh M and Ford P (1989) Nursing rituals, research and rational actions. Butterworth Heinnemann: Oxford.

Wong F, Kember D, Chung L and Yan L (1995) Assessing the level of student reflection from reflective journals. *Journal of Advanced Nursing*, 22: 48–57.

4

Models of Effective and Reflective Teaching and Learning for Best Practice in Clinical Supervision

Dawn Freshwater, Elizabeth Walsh and Philip Esterhuizen

SYNOPSIS

In this chapter, we highlight three different approaches to the introduction of clinical supervision as a concept for promoting good practice using examples from three different settings relating to clinical practice, these being prison services, an acute trust and academia. The text underpins practical examples that are based on learning theory, offering the reader insight into the roles of supervisee and supervisor.

Introduction

Teaching and learning in health care practice has changed dramatically over the past thirty years. The late 1970s and early 1980s heralded the introduction of experiential learning and a more humanistic philosophy underpinning health care and specifically nurse education. This brought about a shift from the didactic nature of classroom instruction to an acknowledgement of the student as an adult learner. The recognition of the value of experiential learning and reflective practice indicates that professional development is a continuous process, acknowledging that knowledge arising from practice has high status, as it has relevance to the delivery of patient care. Part of the challenge for educators has been to create alternative methods of delivering the curriculum that emphasise reflection as both a method of learning and a central tenet of effective and deliberate disciplined practice. This is closely linked with the notion of lifelong learning and autonomous practice.

The introduction of reflective practice and student-centred approaches through experiential learning, while not without their critics, are now central to the development of professional competence and to the integration of learning into practice. The advent of clinical supervision has also, as this text demonstrates, raised many issues not only for practitioners and managers, but also for educators (clinical and academic). In this chapter, we focus on experiential models of teaching and learning the theory and practice of clinical supervision.

It is not our intention to outline a single definitive educational model for the teaching of clinical supervision; we recognize and appreciate that there are a multitude of available training programmes, based on a diversity of educational frameworks. Rather, our aim is to illustrate, through examples, process-oriented ways of facilitating skills training for clinical supervisors. It is worth noting that as Kolb (1984) and others pointed out over two decades ago, learners have individual learning needs and styles and educationalists, therefore, need to allow for a diversity of perceptions, expectations, experiences and evaluations. It is our view that clinical supervision is best learnt through a dynamic and experiential learning process model; thus we describe approaches to teaching and learning the skills of clinical supervision within that educational framework, while demonstrating that there are various structures that can be adapted within even one framework. We emphasise and draw upon a skills-based training through formal academic courses with coursework, teaching and learning using action learning and a non-academic practice-based learning model.

The overarching teaching and learning strategy within the examples that follow is designed to encourage students to engage with supervision in a way that will help them to develop their roles as senior professionals within their field. In addition, the chosen approach means that all participants have equal opportunity to maximise upon the available material and human resources. The strategies aim to foster the skills of reasoned debate and constructive critique through dialogue, presentation and dissemination skills, leadership skills and those of critical reflexivity. A further outcome of the process is for the potential supervisors/supervisees to be able to manage their own learning and become self-directed. This cannot be done without paying close attention to our relationships with others and, as such, relationality is a key concept within the subsequent discussion. The emphasis in this chapter then is on dialogic teaching and learning processes, with participants being encouraged to collaborate and review each other's development. Philosophies of shared principles and collaborative learning are integrated with an appreciation of the individual's learning trajectory within the context of professional practice and their own personal journey.

Teaching and Learning Supervisory Skills: An Action Learning Approach

In the following section, we discuss the use of action learning to support and develop both reflective practice and clinical supervision, using examples based upon research undertaken within HM Prison Service. Two practice development projects that were recently undertaken, in which action learning has been used to support the development and implementation of clinical supervision and reflective practice, will be used to illustrate the benefits and highlight the challenges of using action learning to both teach and develop reflective practice and clinical supervision.

The Prison Context

It is important for the reader to appreciate the context of these projects – that of the prison health service; the cultural context, the learners' understanding and need to develop practice, dictated the approach taken and, as a result, the teaching/ learning approach emerged organically from within the clinical context. The development, implementation and subsequent sustainability of clinical supervision and reflection in the workplace are fraught with barriers and problems; see, for example, Marrow (1997). This is no different in the prison setting, however the barriers and problems do differ and require creative problem solving on behalf of the facilitator (see Freshwater et al., 2001; 2002).

Staff working with prisoners include nurses, prison officers (some with specialist training in health care, catering, suicide prevention, physical education, dog handling, training and education etc.), doctors, sexual health workers, drug and alcohol workers, chiropodists, opticians, pharmacists, teachers, chaplains, probation officers, administrative staff and counsellors to name but a few. It can be seen that the physical, mental, emotional, spiritual and pastoral needs of the prisoner are to be met by a range of professionals working closely together within the prison walls. As such, learning opportunities and training concerning both reflective practice and clinical supervision can assume that where there is prior knowledge it will be diverse and fragmented. The in-house training and professional development of staff working in the prison setting is located within the culture of the prison. It has been noted previously that the culture of the prison affects the ready acceptance of new developments and the learning environment itself; see Walsh (2005) and Freshwater et al. (2002). Crawley (2004) discusses the basic training given to prison officers in terms of its militaristic approach and the focus of training officers to be suspicious. In a recent study, it was found that suspicion and cynicism towards clinical supervision (by both officers and nurses) was rife and even noted as a barrier to its implementation (Freshwater et al., 2002). Further, both the culture of blame and the context of coping in prison health care mitigate against reflective practice, fostering a rather defensive stance, as opposed to the open and trusting stance required for effective clinical supervision.

Reflective Practice and Clinical Supervision

In Chapter 3 of this book, Freshwater suggests that 'clinical supervision and reflective practice are interdependent and inextricably linked through the process of reflection'. As Fowler and Chevannes (1998; p. 380) stated, 'If clinical supervision is seen as a formal system, then reflection appears to be its enabling process.' It is this acceptance and understanding of the link between clinical supervision and reflection that underpinned our use of action learning with prison staff not only to develop reflection but also to implement clinical supervision within the prison setting. A lack of understanding of the nature of clinical supervision within the prison setting and a deep suspicion of it, led us to believe that it would be important for prison staff to appreciate and fully understand the concept and benefits of reflection before clinical supervision would be feasible, as without the ability to reflect on practice, the effective development of clinical supervision would be impossible.

As Musselwhite and colleagues (2005) found the promotion of reflection through action learning successful when working with a multi-disciplinary team in the prison setting on mental health awareness, we adopted this method of teaching, first to promote reflection and subsequently to involve staff in clinical supervision. The theoretical perspective employed is discussed on two levels: first the use of action learning to promote reflection and second the use of action learning to develop clinical supervision.

Using Action Learning to Promote Reflection   Action learning, initially developed by Revans (1980; p. 288) as an approach to training managers in commerce and the public sector, is defined as 'learning by doing with and from others who are also learning by doing'. Similarly McGill and Brockbank (2004; p. 11) describe action learning as 'a continuous process of learning and reflection that happens with the support of a group or "set" of colleagues, with the intention of getting things done'. It is through action learning that participants can utilise their action learning group to discuss new knowledge, develop their skills and initiate change in both the workplace and in their own practice. Action learning therefore promotes the generation of new knowledge through experience that is shared with others. Thus, action learning affords the personal experience centre stage in the learning process while acknowledging the benefits of sharing learning in a social context (McGill and Brockbank, 2004). Clearly, there is a strong link between action learning and reflection, as membership of an action learning group requires its members to engage purposefully in reflection where, by the very nature of action learning, reflection has the potential to unwrap new meaning and understanding. Action learning as a means of supporting reflective and experiential learning is well documented in the literature; see, for example, Graham (1995), Haddock (1997), Heidari and Galvin (2003) and Moon (2004).

The approach used in action learning is distinctly different from traditional, more authoritarian ways of learning in which information is given to individuals to learn in an often solitary and competitive environment (McGill and Brockbank, 2004). By contrast, the emphasis in action learning is on the importance of individual experience, shared within a group, with time and space afforded to group members, allowing them to develop and learn at their own pace in a safe environment. In this sense action learning is closely linked to experiential learning, confluent education and transformational learning (Askew and Carnell, 1998). Action learning is also an opportunity to examine tacit knowledge through reflection and as such, is an ideal mechanism by which to examine the practice of experienced staff. As Bolton (2005; p. 279) stated 'exposing experiences to critical scrutiny in action learning sets can enable individuals to perceive and potentially alter previously taken-for-granted "paradigms" or "stories" which culturally frame aspects of their experience'.

Case Study: The Training of Prison Staff in Mental Health Awareness
Mental health care in prisons has been highlighted as an area for improvement and was identified in the National Service Framework for Mental Health (DoH, 1999) as a priority. In the National Service Framework, it states that local services must explore opportunities to 'improve mental health care for prisoners within existing resources' (DoH, 1999; p. 9). Paton and Jenkins (2002) suggested that this can happen through encouraging the governor and other staff to develop an environment that supports mental health and well-being. In response to this, a training programme in mental health awareness was developed and provided for a group of prison officers and general nurses in one prison where following the training, an action learning group was established, primarily to embed training in practice but which also supported the development of reflective practice (see Figure 4.1). The aim here is not to discuss the course itself, but to examine the nature of the training in terms of the

Module one	Background to understanding mental health and illness
Module two	Mental health awareness • Anxiety disorders • Depression • Bi-polar disorder • Psychosis and schizophrenia • Co-morbidity, substance misuse and mental illness • Personality disorders
Module three	Understanding self harm and suicidal behaviour
Module four	Communication and documentation skills
Module five	Team working and perceived barriers

Figure 4.1 Content of mental health awareness training for prison staff (Musselwhite et al., 2005).

way in which the reflective skills of the staff were developed utilizing action learning.

The training consisted of three days of 'information giving', which while sounding very traditional in terms of the teaching, also included group work and the sharing of experiences. Reflection was therefore undertaken throughout the three days training; however, it is more the nature of the follow-up work done with this group, which is of interest here, as was in this forum that reflection and supervision became central to the participants' development.

Following the initial training, the group met monthly for a period of six months, the primary aim being to help embed theory into practice, discuss experiences and relate them back to the training. Action learning group meetings were also a forum at which the staff could learn from one another, develop their understanding and begin to initiate change back in their workplace. In doing this, it was necessary for the group to develop their skills in reflection as part of their preparation and planning for participation in the meetings. This was addressed in the first action learning group where the facilitator introduced the concept of structured reflection using an example from her own practice, using a structured model of reflection; see Gibbs (1988).

Overall, the action learning aspect of the group was successful with many issues and challenges from the workplace addressed; however, it was the marked increase in the use of reflection that stood out as one of the major benefits to this group and their practice. Through the use of reflection and the subsequent raised professional awareness, group members reported a change in their understanding of mental health in both themselves and in prisoners, and a marked change in their confidence when dealing with prisoners with mental health issues and improvements in their working relationships with colleagues. (This change was evidenced through reflection in the action learning sets, but was also observed by peers among peers.) In this sense the action learning group was an efficient vehicle for the development of reflective skills. This seemed to be particularly related to the group being a safe and supportive environment in which to reflect, an important point raised later in the chapter.

Using Action Learning to Support the Development and Implementation of Clinical Supervision   As has been previously highlighted, action learning promotes learning through experience by sharing that experience with a dedicated group to develop and move on. Action learning to promote reflection was used in one prison to promote reflection as a means to embed previously learnt theory into practice, and to change practice. In contrast to this, action learning is also being used as a way of developing and supporting the implementation of clinical supervision into the prison setting. It is not only nursing staff that benefit from reflection and clinical supervision. Both reflection and clinical supervision can be viewed as significant for all staff working in a caring capacity with prisoners. Indeed, if mentoring and support are viewed as 'caring' then, for the most part, it is the prison officer who is at the forefront of caring for the prisoner. With this in mind, clinical supervision in prison does not just encompass nurses working in the prison environment; there are prison officers with training in health care and prison officers trained in suicide prevention who are also involved in the project outlined next.

Practical Example: The Development of Clinical Supervision in Prison Health Care A United Kingdom Central Council for Nursing, Midwifery and Health Visiting (UKCC) report that examined nursing in secure environments (UKCC and University of Central Lancashire 1999) reached a number of conclusions relevant to the development of clinical supervision in the prison service. It was reported that there was a low level of acceptance of clinical supervision and that clinical supervision was not readily available to nurses working in the prison setting, which tested their professional resilience. They continued 'The patient groups and professional isolation, in some instances would suggest that this is an area where nurses would benefit from the rigorous and systematic application of clinical supervision' (UKCC and University of Central Lancashire, 1999; p. 5).

Following the publication of Nursing in Secure Environments (UKCC and University of Central Lancashire, 1999) and the policy document 'The Future Organisation of Prison Health Care' (NHS Executive/HM Prison Service, 1999) a nationally funded clinical supervision project was commissioned. This project was designed in three phases. Phase one aimed to develop, implement and evaluate clinical supervision appropriate to the needs of prison health care staff. Phase two involved the training of prison staff in clinical supervision incorporating the findings from phase one. Phase three, which is currently in progress at the time of writing, involves the use of regional action learning groups to facilitate a national roll out of clinical supervision. In this phase of the project, regional action learning groups are being used to provide support and supervision in developing clinical supervision throughout England and Wales. Groups of approximately 6–10 staff from a number of prisons in a region meet regularly over the course of 12 months, away from the workplace, with an experienced facilitator to share ideas, and gain support from other group members to implement and sustain clinical supervision in their own prisons.

The 'modus operandi' of the action learning groups is twofold; to provide support in the form of group supervision through the use of an experienced facilitator/supervisor but also to provide action learning for developing and sustaining clinical supervision in practice. This means that the action learning groups, in this context, have a role as both a clinical supervision group, and a role of developing clinical supervision in individual prisons through 'action'. Some major developments have taken place within these groups. Members have discovered and developed new and innovative ways of providing supervision in their own prisons and most notably, in one group, developed a 'toolbox' for their prisons in which examples of best practice in contracts, policies and training materials developed through the action learning group can be found. The 'toolbox' helps to address many of the issues raised through group supervision in terms of implementing clinical supervision and, importantly, has been developed by prison staff, for prison staff and is therefore deemed relevant and useable. Indeed, this action learning group has also begun work on changing terminology, deeming that the term 'clinical supervision' was inappropriate given the inherent custodial, supervisory nature of the prison setting and perceived suspicious culture of its staff. The decision to change the terminology was made as a result of the group feeling that they somehow 'owned' the work they were doing.

These approaches to reflection in clinical supervision, which have been successfully adopted in the prison setting, have, at their core, the concept of action learning. In terms of supporting the development of reflective practice in prison officers, working in a culture used to a more traditional didactic approach to learning and development, action learning has been well received and has made a notable difference to those involved both in terms of their confidence and practice. In supporting the implementation of clinical supervision across the prison estate, action learning appears to be providing the kind of support needed by staff working in the prison environment. A large-scale evaluation at the close of the project will reveal to what extent this approach has been effective; however, interim evaluation and anecdotal evidence at present suggests this model is meeting the needs of the organisation, prison establishments and prison staff.

Strengths and Weaknesses of Action Learning   One of the strengths of using action learning to develop reflective practice and clinical supervision in the prison setting lies in the concept's underpinning philosophy of providing a safe environment in which to share and learn from experience. It is argued that it is the safe environment of action learning groups which, when working in a culture where disclosure is resisted (see Crawley, 2004), provide a haven for sustainable development. With this in mind, however, it must be noted that staff working in a culture where disclosure is opposed, found it difficult to relax and settle into the action learning approach. This issue was addressed very quickly by holding meetings away from the prison setting, out of uniform, with firm ground rules and with facilitators very much aware of the culture and thus able to provide reassurance and understanding.

Attendance at action learning group meetings needs to be consistent and regular. A benefit of using action learning is the improvement in team working that occurs as a result of having consistent attendance. However, ensuring regular attendance can also be a challenge when working with such groups. The ability of prisons to release staff to attend group meetings was initially patchy and as such, much effort was expended in advising managers and group members of the importance of consistency. To meet this challenge time was spent 'building' action learning groups, through working with individuals on a one-to-one basis in the early stages. Although time consuming, this has proved to be a very productive strategy in areas where attendance was an issue. This demonstrates that although action learning can be a very successful approach to developing supervision and reflective practice, it has the risk of being time consuming and labour intensive in terms of both setting up groups and in staff time to attend them.

What follows is a brief SWOT analysis of action learning in developing reflective practice and clinical supervision, (see Figure 4.2), to clarify the benefits of action learning as an effective tool, while acknowledging its limitations. According to Blackwell's Nursing Dictionary, a SWOT analysis is used to 'gauge the strengths and weaknesses of a programme and to survey threats and opportunities' (Freshwater and Maslin-Prothero, 2005; p. 586).

Strengths of action learning	Weaknesses of action learning
• Useful for initiating and sustaining change • Challenges taken-for-granted ideas • Facilitates and develops reflection • Promotes collaborative, multi-disciplinary working	• Time consuming • Resource intensive • Requires strong facilitation • Requires consistent attendance • Requires commitment from members
Opportunities of action learning • Improved staff morale • Clinical supervision provision • Improved ability to reflect both 'on' and subsequently 'in' practice • Improved team working	**Threats to action learning** • Inherent learning culture of organisation • Time constraints • Poor facilitation • Poor understanding by action learning group members • Lack of commitment by organisation and individuals

Figure 4.2 A SWOT analysis of action learning.

In summary, reflective practice is intrinsically developed through action learning as a consequence of the mode of working. From our experiences working with prison staff, who have often presented as initially resistant to this learning approach, the use of a 'neutral' subject about which they are interested proved to be the way in which to develop reflection alongside the main focus of the training, namely mental health awareness. In using this approach, participants are afforded comfort and safety through the structure inherent in traditional training but following this, reflection can be made more overt through the action learning approach. Thus, participants conclude this phase of their development with empirical knowledge generated from training, namely mental health awareness in our case, but also with skills in reflection and an approach to practice underpinned by reflection generated through an action learning framework centred around the original topic.

Clinical supervision is developed through action learning as members receive support through the group, while simultaneously using the action learning component to implement a change, namely clinical supervision. Again, as with initially developing reflexivity in participants through action learning while concentrating on a 'neutral' subject, this approach not only develops skills in reflection, but also generates changes in practice with regard to providing and facilitating clinical supervision in the workplace. The difference here is that the participants involved in the action learning groups are already interested in clinical supervision but have as their aim, the development of systems back in their own establishments. Participation in action learning groups for this group of staff provides a place in which to further their knowledge and receive supervision themselves.

Teaching and Learning Supervisory Skills: A Non-Traditional Practice-Based Approach

In addition to the more traditional mode of delivering training and education, clinical supervision skills are also required by practitioners who are not especially interested in/needing to obtain academic credits but who need, or have an interest in, their use both for their own benefit and for providing clinical supervision for their staff/colleagues. In this example, we define the group of practitioners most likely to follow a non-academic educational programme, going on to discuss the concept of adult learners, the programme content and concluding with reflections on the benefits and limitations of the didactic process. When we use the term non-academic, we do not wish to give the impression that the training is not scholarly, rather to give the sense of a *practice-based programme* which is not beholden to a specified format or structure.

Group Definition and Impact on the Educational Sessions

The example of teaching and learning presented here is based on data collected from a three-day intensive training, commissioned by an acute hospital trust, and based on a training needs analysis. The practitioners that usually engage in this hospital-based training programme have normally followed a work-based educational programme leading to professional qualification and may have undertaken academic post-registration study to achieve a first degree. By definition this group generally consists of practitioners based in practice who have a limited (or sometimes negative) experience of clinical supervision and often of academia; believing they do not have the time to engage in 'non-clinical' activities and who have angst for anything that is apparently academic. Participation in 'non-clinical' learning is of course often mandatory and prescribed by an employing institution, and is sometimes accompanied by feelings of uncertainty and scepticism, although this is usually tempered by an element of interest – either to learn about clinical supervision, or to use the sessions as a platform to articulate disenchantment and discontent related to personal experiences of supervision or academia. The individual sessions spread across the three days can be, and often are, challenging to an educator, who is required to provide meaningful and practical knowledge and skills, while simultaneously dealing with professional and personal baggage, occasionally projected onto the facilitator in the form of a personal attack! In this situation it is imperative that the educator is prepared to interact at whatever level the group presents and is prepared to deal with discussions dynamically and in context. Any unresolved issues may influence group dynamic and process, and if not used appropriately, can sabotage learning and perceptions of safety/trust for the rest of the group (see other chapters in this book for discussions of the significance of trust and safety).

Importantly, the facilitator needs to be mindful of the nature of the group, which consists of adult learners, and draw upon appropriate and relevant educational frameworks. We propose that a confluent education model, strongly based in experiential learning, can be useful when facilitating the teaching and learning of clinical supervision to participants whose focus is on skills acquisition within the practice setting using 'real world' activities. A 'non-academic' approach is important for this group if they are to fully engage in a training programme. Although perceptions differ, there is often an expectation, that time spent learning away from practice is time wasted, which means that the programme needs to be practical and worthwhile. However, as adult learners, the practitioners also need to understand the practicalities of clinical supervision and be open to (if not convinced of and sometimes persuaded!) of its benefits from the start. Many a sceptic has been transformed into a champion for supervision through such facilitation.

Adult Learners and Confluent Education

Over 20 years ago Kolb (1984; p. 50) suggested that 'adults are what they have done', implying that their past experiences were an important starting point for the process of learning. Knowles (1980) also illustrated this in his discussion on dimensions of maturation, noting that adults are primarily involved in a quest for self-actualisation which could mean that, regardless of the participant's apparent motivation, there is an element of self-improvement or self-actualisation underpinning participation in learning (see also Maslow (1968) for a comprehensive understanding of motivations to learn). These two characteristics of adult learners remain important today and have been developed to incorporate and acknowledge the personal process of the individual, more latterly positioning their development in the framework of personal transformation (Johns and Freshwater, 1998; 2005; Freshwater, 2000; Rolfe et al., 2001; Randle, 2002).

Confluent education provides an appropriate educational model and propagates a holistic approach to education. Brown, Phillips and Shapiro (1976) place their ideas of experiential learning in Yeomans' model (Figure 4.3). Starting with an inner area of *intrapersonal* functioning, the individual can be characterised by the different roles and personal attitudes they hold. *Interpersonal* functioning is described as the interaction between the individual and those in their environment, *extrapersonal* functioning – the contexts in which people learn and, all this finally occurs within a matrix of *transpersonal* functioning that forms a philosophical/ spiritual context for the intra/inter/extrapersonal interaction. This all-encompassing concept, while well documented in therapeutic literature, is not specified in other experiential learning models, and can provide a

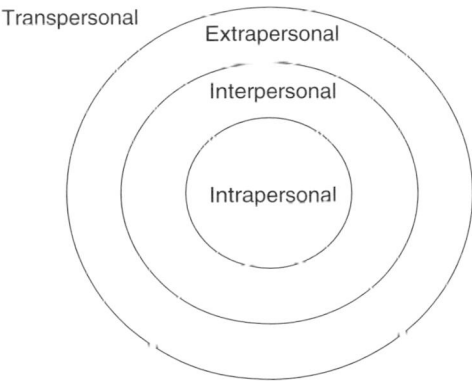

Figure 4.3 Confluent education – Tom Yeomans (Brown, Phillips and Shapiro, 1976).

framework for the educator to explore different areas of functioning with the participants, enabling the individual to link possible mandatory learning with self-actualisation. Interestingly, this model can also be used to examine the processes of clinical supervision, as the practitioner reflects on the personal, the professional, the organisational and the universal aspects of their clinical practice (Freshwater, 2006).

A further characteristic of adult learners is that they are aware of the responsibilities that they carry in their daily work (Bolton, 2005). Castillo (1974) suggested that areas of readiness (to deal with intellectual demands) and responsibility (being able to carry out the tasks required) can be seen as being characteristic for learners who are, at the same time, adult learners and carry responsibility in their daily work. The didactic process needs to address this perception of responsibility and link it to the individual's level of ability to understand and to learn. In other words, the individual's experience is used as a catalyst for the learning process. The essence of confluent education is to blend the physico-psycho-socio-spiritual aspects of being human into a single learning process. The central theme is, therefore, the individual learner's 'Gestalt' where cognitive, affective, readiness and responsibility domains are totally integrated (Castillo, 1974). The confluent educational model described by Castillo (1974) identifies four domains (Figure 4.4) – cognitive (mind), affective (feelings), readiness/awareness and responsibility.

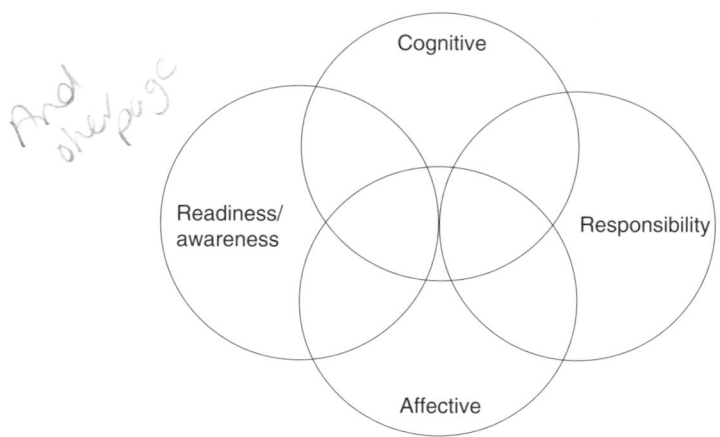

Figure 4.4   The 'four circle' model (Castillo, 1974).

Besides cognitive and affective aspects, Castillo's model allows the educator to isolate important factors and situations in the work environment that affect learning. Castillo suggested that the domains of mind and feelings are directly interrelated both with each other and with the other two domains. It is, however, the individual's degree of readiness/awareness that leads to their being able to carry the responsibility they have. Castillo considered that these two domains do not share a direct interrelationship, but are interrelated via the cognitive and affective domains, thus creating the possibility of integrated learning.

Work-based Learning/Experiential Learning

In an attempt to provide space for the participants to reflect and to integrate the skills and knowledge they develop during the programme, the three study days are spaced, ideally, a week apart. Participants are invited to use work-related vignettes and case studies, past or present, during the learning process. The interactive sessions take the form of different types of supervision during which the participants' situations are discussed. By using this approach, the participants are exposed to the experience and value of clinical supervision directly related to their daily work. Furthermore as this group of participants relies on practical experience, the idea of role play as a teaching method is often even more angst-invoking and seen as being 'non-reality'. The approach of using actual work situations in 'simulated' clinical supervision sessions overcomes the concept of role play, but naturally requires that the group commit to confidentiality and participation at the outset – this exposure provides them with a personal experience of understanding the need to perceive safety and identify their feelings of vulnerability. In this way the participant becomes acutely aware of their individual contribution to a clinical supervision session, and simultaneously group processes and dynamics – embracing multiple loop learning as proposed by Greenwood (1998) and Lingsma and Scholten (2001).

The three study days are planned as full days and the participants are invited to think about their understanding of clinical supervision but are not provided with background reading as preparation to the sessions. Although a full day's session provides space and scope for discussion, the facilitator should be aware of the group dynamic and level of concentration as this type of practitioner often finds it difficult to remain engaged in a classroom setting for such a long time – highlighting the need for a high degree of interactive facilitation. Due to the practical nature of the background of the participants the theoretical concepts underpinning clinical supervision is spread across the three days and clearly and directly related to the experience and understanding in the group. This theory emerges from the practice exemplars defined by the group participants.

Experience demonstrates that practitioners often enter an educational session thinking they know little or nothing about the subject matter. By using Socratic Dialogue to provoke and stimulate (this process is comprehensively described by Todd, 2005) the group is encouraged to share their ideas and knowledge, and enter into discussion with one another – the facilitator leads the discussion and poses questions allowing the participants to name and discuss all relevant issues.

Theoretical information is presented as a summary, incorporating new ideas not raised by the group; in this way participants are directly able to receive feedback on their level of knowledge. This approach links with the notion of conscientisation (education being an empowering and emancipatory process), rather than a passive consumption of information on the part of the participant (Freire, 1970; Freshwater, 2000). To remain congruent with this philosophical approach, seminar-type work in which the educator presents information in a lecture format is kept to a minimum. At this point it is also important to note that experiential learning has fairly major implications for group size which should ideally be between 12 and 20. A larger group is difficult to manage for a single facilitator and is a deterrent to active participation and is a threat to safety.

In brief, day one is spent on introductions, offering the participants space to articulate their expectations and learning objectives for the three days and their experiences in the area of clinical supervision. Often participants verbalise anxieties and negative experiences at this time and it is important that the facilitator takes the time to allow sharing and facilitates group discussion on the issues being presented. This helps to develop a feeling of safety and confidentiality with the group and provides a foundation for the group activities planned during the course of the three study days. It also provides an opportunity for the facilitator to suggest that some situations, presented by the group members, could be used as vignettes during the group activity and allows the facilitator to introduce the concept of interactive group activity outside the realms of role play.

The fact that the group's experiences are being taken seriously and that the individual is being offered a platform to deconstruct real situations generally results in engagement and commitment of the participants.

CLINICAL SUPERVISION EDUCATION – DAY 1

- Introductions
- Personal experience of supervision
- Defining supervision
- Different types of supervision
- Skills practice: One-on-one supervision
- Evaluation of course objectives
- Develop individual audit of skills
- Reflect on personal skills in individual supervision

Once the group dynamic has been set informally, discussion within the group usually flows spontaneously. To stimulate cohesiveness within the group and allow the participants to re-establish their comfort zone, smaller groups are formed and the groups are requested to enter into discussion, reach consensus and formulate a definition of clinical supervision. Each group in turn presents their definition which is written up on a flip chart by the facilitator. Using the definitions presented by the group the facilitator leads a group discussion to identify the ideas and assumptions within the group and attempts to deconstruct them. A number of published definitions are presented and the group is asked to critique them and choose one to serve as a foundation for the three days. By defining supervision in this way the facilitator is able to introduce theoretical concepts and a variety of theoretical definitions.

The rationale behind this approach is to stimulate active engagement, introduce theoretical concepts; illustrate the subjectivity of theory and, therefore stimulate the critical use of evidence-based practice; provide insight into levels of individual knowledge and assumptions; and create cohesiveness and safety within the group. A natural progression for the group is to participate in the first clinical supervision exercise as the group members are in a communicative mode and already subdivided into smaller groups. The participants are, ideally, divided into groups of three – a supervisor, a supervisee and an observer and, after a brief explanation on the types of clinical supervision the groups are invited to attempt a one-on-one supervision session basing it on the definition they had chosen previously. The role of the observer is to provide feedback on whether the session is consistent with the definition. The rationale behind this activity is to create a situation where a shared experience of supervision occurs and to link this to theoretical concepts.

Structure, advice and further theoretical frameworks that link to the participants' concrete experience are introduced as appropriate. An aspect generally raised by the participants in the debriefing session after the exercise is their shared experience of vulnerability. Using this experience the concept of confidentiality and safety is introduced. The participants are invited to establish and agree on the rules they wish to have in place for the three days and this forms the basis for a discussion on confidentiality and a supervision agreement/ contract which is dealt with in more detail on the third day. The one-on-one exercise is repeated three times throughout the rest of the first day with the participants forming new groups for each exercise. More structure and information is provided during the debriefing session following each exercise and includes a discussion on the differences between supervision and counselling and how to identify and set boundaries both from a supervisor's and supervisee's perspective. By the end of the day each participant should have had the opportunity to fulfil each of the three roles of supervisor, supervisee and observer. The first day concludes with the participants evaluating the objectives they had set in the morning and reflecting on how far they have come in achieving them, but also offering them the opportunity to re-define their objectives and make them more concrete where appropriate. At this stage the participants are provided with a number of background articles and requested to read them in preparation for the second session.

Day two commences with reflection and time is allotted for discussion around participants' experiences of the first day or experiences and insights possibly gained in the course of the intervening week. Time is also allotted for discussion and questions related to the literature provided at the end of the first day. Using the participants' experience of and reflections on the one-on-one supervision exercise on the first day the role and responsibility of the supervisor and supervisee are discussed and supported with literature. The insight gained by this discussion is linked to potential pitfalls focussing on the role of the supervisor.

CLINICAL SUPERVISION EDUCATION – DAY 2

– Reflections on previous day and discussion
– Role definition supervisor/supervisee in relation to type of supervision
– Pitfalls of supervision – focussing on the role of the supervisor
– Skills practice: Group supervision I ('Open agenda' peer group supervision)
– Evaluation of course objectives
– Develop individual audit of skills
– Reflect on personal skills in group supervision

Information is provided on different forms of clinical supervision and the strengths and weaknesses of individual and group supervision. This information provides an introduction to the first peer group supervision exercise in which participants form smaller groups of +/- 5 members for an exercise using an 'open agenda' peer group supervision. In this exercise one group member volunteers to be supervisee and the rest of the members provide supervision within an allotted time. The exercise is concluded with a plenary discussion on the benefits and pitfalls of the session. The participants are encouraged to reflect on how they could improve their activity using the theory as criteria and to identify what they would need to develop if they are to contribute to the session using a reflective model (in this case Driscoll, 2001; see Driscoll and Teh, 2001) is used as it provides a clear step in focussing on a selected aspect of the situation. During this discussion issues related to personal and professional boundaries and supervision versus counselling often arise. This exercise is repeated three times in the course of the second day and the participants are encouraged to form a new group configuration for each exercise. The rationale behind this is to expose the participants to different group dynamics and allow them to build relationships with the group members, thereby helping them to establish a network across the organisation. The second day concludes with the participants re-evaluating the objectives they had set initially and reflecting on whether they had achieved them. As on the first day, this activity again offers the opportunity for the participants to re-define their objectives and make them more concrete where appropriate. The rationale here is that participants become aware of their learning being an ongoing cycle and that their objectives need continual evaluation and re-defining.

The participants are encouraged to refer to the background articles provided on the first day, to re-read them critically and to bring points of discussion to the third day. On day 3, the course aims to provide further practical exercises in group reflection, with additional opportunities to discuss the organisational aspects of clinical supervision. This session, once again, commences with reflection on the participants' experience of days 1 and 2, situations involving communication that they identified in the work situation and any issues relating to the literature they may want to discuss. Using this input a link can be made to organisational preconditions that need to be in place and challenges that may arise when attempting to introduce clinical supervision for staff. Participants, at this stage, often discuss personal issues and situations they have experienced similar to those discussed on the first day – only the discussion generally now takes a more constructive and proactive form rather than the emotive, reactionary response articulated initially.

CLINICAL SUPERVISION EDUCATION – DAY 3

– Reflections on previous day and discussion
– Levels of supervision/defining objectives for a supervision session
– What needs to be in place for supervision to work?
– What might prevent supervision from working well?
– Formulating questions in supervision
– Pitfalls of supervision – focussing on the role of the supervisee
– Drawing up a supervision agreement/contract
– Setting boundaries
– Recording sessions
– Skills practice: Group supervision II ('Reflection on own role' peer group supervision)
– Develop individual audit of skills
– Reflect on personal skills in individual and group supervision
– Plans to take supervision forward
– Evaluation of course objectives

This changed attitude is an opportune moment to introduce the role and responsibility of the supervisee and to commence with a second peer group supervision exercise. The participants again form groups consisting of $+/-$ 5 persons. For the second exercise the group elects a supervisee who describes an issue without interruption with the exception of a few questions from the rest of the group at the end to clarify issues, if appropriate. The supervisee then disengages from the group and listens as the group discusses what they would have done/how they would have perceived the situation. After listening to the discussion the supervisee shares how their perception has (not) changed and how they intend addressing the issue. The groups re-convene for a plenary discussion on the strengths and weaknesses of this type of clinical supervision.

Using a reflective model the participants are encouraged to reflect on how they could improve their activity as supervisor and supervisee to attain optimal benefit from the supervisory session. This exercise is repeated a second time and the participants are encouraged to work in a different group configuration. Towards the end of day 3 the issues of supervision agreements and contracts, including the ethics of keeping records of the sessions, transparency and monitoring outcomes are addressed. This is generally done by critiquing existing examples of supervision agreements and adapting an agreement to suit the needs of the group. During the discussion on agreements, the participants generally move spontaneously onto discussing how they intend taking supervision sessions forward and it becomes apparent how networks have been established within the group. The rationale behind the third day focuses strongly on analysis and critique as it is now that the participants need to make informed decisions about the use of supervision models and contracts.

In conclusion the participants are invited to evaluate the product and process of the three days in terms of their set objectives, their initial expectations, the teaching and learning strategies and the learning environment. The participants are requested to formulate a plan of action to take away with them as to how they intend developing their skills and implementing clinical supervision sessions.

Benefits and Limitations

With regard to limitations, currently, the most apparent is that there is a total lack of follow-up after completion of the three days; this is linked to who should be taking responsibility for implementing and sustaining change through adequate support. Although the participants have set up a network system, they will naturally face organisational challenges and peer resistance and as such it is questionable whether they will have sufficient know-how and resilience to manage the implementation of their skills. Although insight into personal and professional limitations is a positive characteristic, some participants enter the three-day sessions with the goal of establishing clinical supervision for their staff. However, on completion of the three days some participants come to the realisation that they need to build their own experience by participating in peer supervision sessions prior to implementing clinical supervision for others. A delay in establishing clinical supervision sessions according to the original plan may result in managers negating the value of the educational programme.

The main benefit of this type of practice-based programme is similar to those already identified through action learning, that is, it is directly related to the participant's work experience and acknowledges the starting point of the learner. By approaching teaching from a confluent education perspective, the domains of 'readiness/awareness' and 'responsibility' provide neutral starting points for discussion that are then addressed via the cognitive and affective domains. This approach appears to be non-threatening to the participant but, at the same time, provides the educator with sufficient practice-related material to introduce theoretical concepts without undue participant stress or resistance. Furthermore, it allows participants to take part in reflection and clinical supervision in action and to experience benefits these interventions can have.

The experience also highlights the importance of confidentiality and peer support. As the theoretical, ethical and organisational aspects of clinical supervision are presented within the context of the participants' work and are provided in a way that allows the participant to link the new information directly to their perceived needs, the information can be used directly and is perceived to be appropriate and usable. Participants are exposed to different models of supervision during the educational days and are, therefore, able to gauge the model's benefits and limitations. This insight allows the individual to make an informed choice as to the most appropriate model to be used in specific situations. The experience of working with different models of clinical supervision also allows the participant to identify areas of learning that they may need to address, either as a supervisee or a supervisor. Other benefits include the fact that participants have the opportunity of networking with others and building collaborative relationships across departments and disciplines, and to develop an understanding of the organisational preconditions needed to implement clinical supervision. Although having chosen to follow a programme that does not provide academic accreditation, participants value receiving a certificate of attendance to be included in their portfolio and evaluation indicates a pride in their achievements during the three-day sessions.

Teaching and Learning Supervisory Skills: The Traditional Academic Module

The programme that is referred to here was developed as part of an academic modular framework that allowed practitioners to undertake supervisory training as either a stand alone module, or as part of a degree pathway. Delivered over a period of 12 weeks students joining the programme spent a total of 7 days in face to face contact and were engaged in skills practice in their own clinical setting in between scheduled teaching time. The clinical supervision module not only provided an important forum for the testing of ideas and the critical appraisal of students' work drawn from clinical practice, but also an opportunity to examine parallel processes between supervisor and supervisee through experiential learning processes (see e.g. Freshwater, 2000; Rolfe et al., 2001). Reflective practice was central to the integration of theory and practice and as such understanding of reflection and models of reflective practice were debated early on in the module (see Chapter 3 on reflection and supervision in this book). The module was based on a policy that supported independent study through collaborative relationships, providing an evidence-based infrastructure that is a necessary part of any successful professional programme.

As part of the programme careful consideration was given as to whether guided reflection through clinical supervision is essentially an educational technique within a learning culture or whether in fact it is the learning culture itself. As Johns (2005) recently observed, this consideration is crucial, not least because it reflects a paradigm clash between theory-led teaching and practice-led learning. He noted that:

> As an educational technique, reflection would be used alongside other teaching techniques governed by the teacher's agenda. As a

learning culture, reflection is the core around which spins information systems to inform the process of learning through everyday experience governed by the practitioner's agenda.

Given the extensive detail of the previous examples, we do not wish to repeat information related to the content and the delivery of the same, rather we have provided two examples of individual teaching sessions which while indicating the content, also provide a sense of the more formal links between this module and the academic institution within which it was facilitated (see Figures 4.5 and 4.6). The main difference in the delivery and development of this more formal academic approach to the teaching and learning of clinical supervision relates to the use of practical and theoretical assignments.

An example of a theoretical assignment is presented below, readers should be aware that we are not suggesting that this is the best way to approach assessing theoretical knowledge of learning, rather we use it as an illustration of the ways in which formal learning of clinical supervision can be assessed. However, it is also worth noting the relationship between the practitioner's own clinical practice and the application and utility of literature/evidence. Once again, the integration of theory and practice through experience becomes the foci of the learning. One of the central tenets of the programme is that of transformational learning, in which theory, research and practice merge into a praxis oriented understanding of the inter-relationship of differing ways of knowing. To this end students are guided through a process which loosely follows four distinct stages (well enunciated by Poincare (1952 cited in Neville, 1989) and Wallas (1926 cited in Neville, 1989), developed by Neville (1989) and further refined by Askew and Carnell (1998), Freshwater (1998; 2000) and Parker (2002)). These being:

- An initial investigation termed the *preparation*
- A period of rest known as the *incubation*
- The occurrence of a sudden and *illuminatory* solution
- Finally conscious rational development of understanding to validate the insight-*verification*.

Those of you who have had to complete a written assignment will be aware of the cyclical movement between these stages as new knowledge is percolating, digesting and being reconstructed to sit with our own norms, values, beliefs and indeed our personal

Title of session	Advanced beginner to expert and clinical supervisor

Relationship to other sessions
Relates to evidence-based practice and implementation of clinical supervision.

Duration of session 3 hours

Learning outcomes
To clarify the role of the Supervisor in facilitating expert practice.
To examine the stages of development in the role of Clinical Supervisor using the parallel process of nursing practice.

Key content
In pairs explore own experience of developing a skill outside nursing. What were the stages you went through? How did you know when you had got where you wanted to be?
Look at model of competence:
Unconscious incompetence
Conscious incompetence
Conscious competence
Unconscious competence
The role of intuition in Clinical Supervision.
The expert nurse as conscious of their incompetence.
Is there an expert?

Recommended teaching strategies
Student experience, working in pairs
Small group discussion
Some didactic input from tutor

Required resources
Handouts
Flipchart

Associated student study activities
Reading from Journal Club
Own experience

Recommended reading
Rolfe, G. (1998) Beyond Expertise. In Johns, C. and Freshwater, D. (1998) *Transforming Nursing Through Reflective Practice*
Benner P. (1984) *From Novice to Expert*, California: Addison Wesley
Schon D. A. (1987) *The Reflective Practitioner*, San Francisco: Jossey Bass

Figure 4.5 Summary of teaching session.

102

Title of session   Clinical supervision and evidence-based practice

---

Relationship to other sessions
Fundamental to the whole notion of Clinical Supervision and Reflective Practice and to the development of evidence-based practice

---

Duration of session 3 hours

Learning outcomes
To have a deeper understanding of how Reflection and Clinical Supervision interface with research in nursing practice.
To be able to relate Clinical Supervision to clinical effectiveness and clinical governance.

Key content
What is professional knowledge?
Use of photographs to stimulate debate.
Who is the most professional nurse?
Who is most effective? In professional/public eye?
What is effective practice?
Two approaches to practice – parallel process.
Two approaches to Clinical Supervision.
Competency based versus philosophy based.
Relate to the professionalisation of nursing and making private knowledge/public.
Issues of evaluating nursing – who is the best person to measure nurses?

Recommended teaching strategies
Experiential
Small group discussion
Some didactic input

Required resources
OHP
Flipchart
Handouts
Student experience

Associated student study activities
Own experience
Reading from Journal Club

Figure 4.6   Summary of teaching session.

experience. However, we also undergo similar processes when learning a new skill such as supervision.

Case Example: Theoretical Assignment

Rationale The aim of this assignment is to:

- Explore the current developments in clinical supervision in your own area of practice;
- To make judgements about the literature and its contribution to your current practice;
- To use reflective skills to critically read and analyse the literature/research in relation to the module and your own experience.

Developing a Work Plan You are required to prepare a plan of work and present this to your personal tutor for discussion. The plan of work should include the following:

- The rationale for your choice of literature review and its relevance to your practice.
- The main issues to be addressed.
- A summary of how the review is to be developed.
- List of key references based on a preliminary literature search.

You are required to select three articles written in the field of clinical supervision that relate to your own area of practice; where relevant literature is limited you are advised to seek advice from your facilitator. Having read and interpreted the literature you are expected to discuss within your review how the literature relates to your own understanding and development of what is happening in clinical supervision in you own practice. It is expected that you will refer to the learning from the module and your own personal experience. You should inform the reader of the data sources you consulted when undertaking the search, and the results of your search including the amount of literature available on the topic. When addressing the abundance or limitations of literature identified within your search, you should refer to the implications for current and future developments in nursing practice. Please submit with your assignment copies of your chosen articles.

Benefits and Limitations

The benefits and limitations of undertaking a formal academic module in clinical supervision are numerous, but these mainly relate to the location of the course within an academic institution and an academic framework, such as a degree pathway. Benefits include access to a wide range of educational resources; acknowledgement and accreditation of prior learning; formally recognised qualification that can be built on; learning takes place in a neutral environment away from clinical practice and there is the opportunity to meet a wide variety of participants. Nevertheless, such educational systems can tend to be somewhat constraining in terms of the structure of programmes and their delivery, although more flexible methods of learning are now being developed. Requirements for attendance and contribution are often more formally measured in academic settings and can be closely linked to assessment, which might seem at first glance to be in direct opposition to the philosophy of adult learning.

Conclusion

From an epistemological standpoint the type of knowing and learning that we have provided examples of in this chapter is in the domain of experiential knowledge. That is, knowledge gained through direct personal encounter with a person or subject; it is knowledge gained through relationship and what critical theorists refer to as critical or emancipatory knowledge (Habermas, 1972; Fay, 1987). This is particularly important given the contexts that we have described. We posit that experiential personal knowing can provide the bridge between which propositional and practical knowledge, can flow. Experiential ways of learning can act as the tools for building a bridge between theory and practice, leading to a more integrated knowing in action. We suggest that experiential frameworks are appropriate ways for preparing practitioners for their role as supervisors and for supporting them in their practice. As we have highlighted, this approach features reflection on practice as a key component of learning and a student (practitioner) centred, facilitative, non-directive approach to teaching is adopted. It is also what might be termed a 'deep' approach to learning (Freshwater, 2000). The learning that takes place in the deep approach is one in which formal learning is integrated with personal experience to develop an understanding of meaning. Motivation for deep learning is essentially intrinsic, although learning is made concrete through the interplay of the inner and the outer. Deep learning is, however, associated with challenging the familiar and is often accompanied or impelled by discomfort (Joyce, 1984; Askew and Carnell, 1998; Freshwater, 2000). This may account for some of the resistance to experiential learning and indeed to clinical supervision, which also aims to challenge the familiar. We wish to end by signifying the importance of creativity and fun in the teaching and learning of clinical supervision. We believe, as do many others that ... 'any education that in any way neglects imagination is an education that results in a sociopathic society of manipulators. We learn how to deal with others and become a society of dealers' (Neville, 1989; p. 171). *We are not dealers, we are carers, and any training, including that of clinical supervision needs to hold this as a fundamental aspect of the teaching and learning process.*

References

Askew S and Carnell E (1998) *Transformatory Learning: Individual and Global Change*. Cassell, London.

Bolton G (2005) Taking responsibility for our stories: in reflective practice, action learning and Socratic dialogue. *Teaching in Higher Education*, 10 (2): 271–280.

Brown GI, Phillips M and Shapiro SB (1976) *Getting it All Together: Confluent Education*. The Phi Delta Kappa Educational Foundation, Indiana.

Castillo G (1974) *Left-handed Teaching*. Prager Publishers, New York.

Crawley E (2004) *Doing Prison Work*. Willan Publishing, Devon.

DoH (1999) National Service Framework for Mental Health: Modern Standards and Service Models. HMSO London.

Driscoll J and Teh B (2001). The potential of reflective practice to develop individual orthopaedic nurse practitioners and their practice. *Journal of Orthopaedic Nursing*, 5: 95–103.

Fay B (1987) *Critical Social Science*. Polity Press, Cambridge.

Fowler J and Chevannes M (1998) Evaluating the efficacy of reflective practice within the context of clinical supervision. *Journal of Advanced Nursing*, 27: 379–382.

Freire P (1970) *Pedagogy of the Oppressed*. Penguin, London.

Freshwater D (1998) The Philosopher's Stone. In: Johns C and Freshwater D (eds) *Transforming Nursing Through Reflective Practice*. Blackwell Science Oxford Ch 9.

Freshwater D (2000) *Transformatory Learning in Nurse Education.* Nursing Praxis International, Southsea.

Freshwater D, Walsh L and Story L (2002) Prison health care: Developing leadership through clinical supervision. *Nursing Management,* 8 (9): 16–20.

Freshwater D and Maslin-Prothero S (eds) (2005) *Blackwell's Nursing Dictionary.* Blackwell, Oxford.

Freshwater D, Walsh L and Story L (2001) Prison health care: Developing leadership through clinical supervision. *Nursing Management,* 8 (8): 10–13.

Gibbs G (1988) *Learning By Doing: A Guide to Teaching and Learning Methods,* Further Education Unit, Oxford Brookes University, Oxford.

Graham I (1995) Reflective practice: using the action learning group mechanism. *Nurse Education Today,* 15: 28–32.

Greenwood (1998) The role of reflection in single and double loop learning. *Journal of Advanced Nursing,* 27: 1048–1053.

Habermas J (1972) *Knowledge and Human Interest.* Heinnemann, London.

Haddock J (1997) Reflection in groups: contextual and theoretical considerations within nurse education and practice. *Nurse Education Today,* 17: 381–385.

Heidari F and Galvin K (2003) Action learning groups: can they help students develop their knowledge and skills? *Nurse Education in Practice,* 3: 49–55.

Johns C (2005) In: Johns C and Freshwater D (eds) *Transforming Nursing Through Reflective Practice.* 2nd ed. Blackwell Science, London.

Johns C and Freshwater D (1998) *Transforming Nursing Through Reflective Practice.* Blackwell Science, Oxford.

Joyce BR (1984) Dynamic disequilibrium: the intelligence of growth. *Theory into Practice,* 23 (1): 26–34.

Knowles MS (1980) *The Modern Practice of Adult Education: From Pedagogy to Andragogy,* Prentice Hall, Engelwood Cliffs, New Jersey.

Kolb D (1984) *Experiential Learning.* Prentice Hall, Engelwood-Cliffs, New Jersey.

Lingsma M and Scholten M (2001) Coachen op competentie-ontwikkeling. Soest: H. Nelissen.

Marrow CE (1997) Promoting reflective practice through structured clinical supervision. *Journal of Advance Nursing,* 5: 77–82.

Maslow AH (1968, 1999) *Towards a Psychology of Being.* John Wiley and Sons, New York.

McGill I and Brockbank A (2004) *The Action Learning Handbook.* Routledge Falmer, London.

Moon JA (2004) *A Handbook of Reflective and Experiential Learning.* Routledge Falmer, London.

Musselwhite C, Walsh E and Freshwater D (2005) Evaluation of Mental Health Awareness Training: A Case Study at HMP High Down.

Neville B (1989) *Understanding Psyche.* Collins Dove, Australia.

NHS Executive and HM Prison Service (1999) *The Future Organisation of Prison Health Care*. Department of Health, London.

Parker M (2002) In: Freshwater D (ed.) *Therapeutic Nursing: Improving Patient Care Through Reflection*. Sage, London.

Paton J and Jenkins R (eds) (2002) *Mental Health Primary Care in Prison*. Royal Society of Medicine, London.

Randle J (2002) The shaping of moral identity and practice. *Nurse Education in Practice*, 2: 251–256.

Revans R (1980) *Action Learning: New Techniques for Management*. Blond and Briggs, London.

Rolfe G, Freshwater D and Jasper M (2001) *Critical Reflection for Nursing and the Caring Professions: A User's Guide*. Palgrave, Basingstoke

Todd G (2005) In: Johns C and Freshwater D (eds) *Transforming Nursing Through Reflective Practice*. 2nd Ed. Blackwell Publishing, Oxford, Ch 3.

UKCC and University of Central Lancashire (1999) *Nursing in Secure Environments*. UKCC, London

Walsh L (2005) Developing prison health care through reflective practice. In: Johns C and Freshwater D (eds) *Transforming Nursing Through Reflective Practice*. Blackwell Publishing, Oxford

5

Critical Reflection and Clinical Supervision: Facilitating Transformation

Brendan McCormack and Liz Henderson

SYNOPSIS

In this chapter, we present an account of a practice development programme with clinical nurse specialists (CNS) in a cancer and palliative care service of a large teaching hospital. The development programme was set within principles of clinical supervision and action learning, but did not try to apply a particular model of supervision and learning. A conceptual framework was developed based on methodological principles derived from critical social science and structured around three action cycles – developing a shared *vision* for the project and the CNS role; understanding the *culture and context* of care; developing *leadership* to effect practice change. The chapter describes the development of facilitation skills of the lead facilitator and of participants and an analysis of the journey of learning and development that participants underwent. We conclude that establishing mechanisms for systematically developing, narrating and analysing shared practice stories can be an enlightening process in its own right and can add much to our understanding of the processes used and the outcomes experienced.

Introduction

> It was safe before you came along. Now it's all messy. I keep on seeing problems in the way I practice. Why weren't they there

before? You tell me to feel good about my work, but how can I when all I can see is dross. (excerpt from Brendan's reflective diary)

Opening our eyes to the reality of our practice is always a painful process (if it is to be meaningful!). Seeing what is there and going beyond the obvious is a key challenge in the development of practice. Clinical supervision represents one mechanism for 'going beyond the obvious' and exploring the deeper aspects of 'self' in the context of effective practice. It is widely acknowledged that understanding 'self' is key to transformative action. In this chapter, we present an overview of clinical supervision in the context of facilitating transformation of 'self'. A two-year practice development programme, designed to enable Clinical Nurse Specialists (CNS) maximize their role potential, will be outlined. The shared journey undertaken by the CNS and Liz as programme facilitator provides an opportunity for gaining greater insight into the processes used and the impact of the development activities.

In this chapter, we begin by making some observations about clinical supervision and developing practice. We then describe the practice context and background to the project that Liz facilitated, outline the methodology and development frameworks used, narrate the group story and report the project outcomes. Finally, we will consider the implications of such work for the development of practice and practitioners.

Clinical Supervision and Transformation

Clinical supervision is a movement that has been in existence for some time. In nursing at least, a large body of 'clinical supervision' literature exists. Since its high profile formal introduction in nursing in the 1990s, interest in clinical supervision in a variety of professional groupings (nursing, midwifery and social work, for example) has continued. This interest is significant as it reflects a sustained interest among practitioners to develop their internal motivations for providing quality approaches to practice – motives that may have brought them into their chosen profession in the first place, but have often been lost in the organisational systems of work. Such an interest is indeed welcomed as the dilemma of the contemporary professional practitioner working in a predominantly postmodernist society lies in the fact that the body of knowledge used and the expectations of society served are changing so rapidly.

In much of the contemporary policy and strategic literature it is increasingly recognised that the reality of practice is as Schön (1991) described – messy, complex and enmeshed in ethical conflict. Practice is contextually located and embedded in multiple cultures that are created and re-created by the 'actors' within that context. Individuals can influence the context of practice but this influence can only be translated into sustainable change when the culture is receptive to it (Argyris, 1999). Cultural change happens from 'within' and Manley (2004) refers to this as 'workplace culture', that is, the multiple cultures that make up the setting of practice (i.e. the workplace or context). Accessing these cultures enables the release of the practice knowledge that is embedded in experience, contextually bound and rarely reproduced in propositional form (Titchen and Higgs, 2001). Embracing such reality of practice treats nurses as adult learners, set within the underpinning belief that adults learn what 'they need to learn' and what makes sense to their experience (Schon, 1991). This approach values knowledge that is both inductively and deductively derived (Kitson et al., 1998).

Clinical supervision emphasises the building on knowledge generated through practice experiences. 'Experience' is seen as a valuable source of knowledge. Recognising and learning from the development of nurses' experience in a particular practice context is considered to be an essential route towards the development of 'expertise' in practice (Benner et al., 1996; Manley, 2000; McCormack and Titchen, 2001). While debates exist about the most appropriate model of clinical supervision for practice, the reality is that there is little evidence to indicate the 'ideal' model. However, whatever the model of supervision in place, we can suggest that some principles should underpin the model chosen if it is to be effective in bringing about change. The model should:

- Utilise processes that are negotiated and that are an integral component of practice development.
- Focus on personal and professional effectiveness.
- Enable the systematic development of 'self' as practitioner and 'self' in the context of person-centred practice.
- Integrate reflexive approaches to the evaluation of the effectiveness of structures, processes and outcomes.
- Consider knowledge to be contextually bound and therefore new knowledge is derived from an engagement with the context of everyday practice.

From working with practitioners however, we know that practitioners do not find it easy to talk in a meaningful way about the 'everyday' work that is done with others. Thus, creating connections between what is discussed in supervision and bringing about changes in the cultures of practice is difficult and challenging. Indeed, the complexity associated with demonstrating practice outcomes from reflective practice, clinical supervision and action learning, (for example), is often a key challenge in an outcomes driven health care world. While the rhetoric of person-centred practice prevails (McCormack, 2004) the reality is that measurement of effectiveness in health care delivery continues to focus on numbers treated, waiting times, waiting lists and length of hospital stay. Outcomes such as meeting the needs of distressed patients who are in pain, elderly patients who cannot return to their home, immobile patients who can no longer defecate without assistance, relatives who experience distress at being unable to continue to care for their partner and nursing colleagues who do not know how to cope with such emotional work continue to be given less priority than the 'hard' outcomes of health care. Integrating these person-centred outcomes with organisational priorities is a key challenge that we have to meet in establishing developmental frameworks in health care settings.

Wilson et al. (2005) highlighted the challenges of changing practice culture in settings that espouse person-centred values. A variety of models were needed to bring about meaningful change that was sustainable. Fundamentally, the work undertaken by Wilson et al. (2005) demonstrated the importance of providing opportunities for nurses and others to re-articulate their central values in caring, make them visible and find ways of transforming the workplace culture to make these espoused caring values 'real'. Clinical supervision is one such model that can be used for transforming workplace cultures. However, it is evident that despite a sustained focus on clinical supervision in nursing for more than ten years, its implementation continues to be patchy and there continues to be suspicion among many nurses about its focus and intent. Perhaps therefore, the focus should be less on the naming of a particular model and more on achieving clarity in organisations about the type of culture that is needed for effective person-centred practice. Cultures where learning is an explicit component of practice and where there are formal systems and processes in place to enable learning from experience. Systems and processes that systematically assist nurses to reflect on practice experience, critically review the elements of that practice, actively engage in developing/experimenting with practice and synthesising the learning gained from the process.

For these cultures to be created, criticism need not be suppressed (as a threat or an act of blaming) but is instead welcomed as a part of a continuous learning process. However, creating open rather than suppressive cultures requires what Freshwater (2000) and others (Jackson et al., 2002; McKenna et al., 2003) have referred to as the need to eliminate 'abusive cultures' characterised by horizontal violence. Instead, cultures that require what Winter and Munn-Giddings (2001) refer to as an 'emotional climate' need to be created, that is, the nature of relationships and interactions among and between staff groups. Goleman (1996) refers to this as 'emotional intelligence' – the art of supportive criticism, emotional self-awareness, respecting diversity of opinion as a resource rather than a personal threat, listening to and learning from each other and maintaining group productivity. Operationalising this emotional intelligence requires group/team members to listen to each other as equal partners, explicitly appreciate each other's contributions, value diversity of opinion and acknowledge individual and group feelings as an important part of practice.

The development model in place should lead to meaningful action – actions that are instigated and owned by practitioners and supported by service leaders at every level. Knowledge generated externally (e.g. from academic communities, professional bodies and statutory organisations) would be welcomed in that it would help to place local developments in a strategic context. Creating such a culture does not (in the first instance) require the establishment of 'new' structures. However, it does require processes to be put in place that clarify and make explicit values underpinning practice, embrace transformational leadership, clarify roles among leaders and 'enablers' of cultural change and that are systematically and rigorously operationalised. Evaluation of practice should not rely solely on managerial driven agendas of efficiency and effectiveness to demonstrate corporate accountability. Instead, evaluation should be seen as 'self-evaluation' utilising a variety of approaches including feedback from colleagues, from service users and from service leaders in a continuous cycle of improvement.

It can be argued that clinical supervision, supported reflective practice and action learning are formalised processes for developing such cultures of inquiry and enabling practitioners to develop emotional intelligence. However, we would argue that any or all of these models need to be integrated into a developmental framework that has an explicit intent of 'transformation' that is negotiated and rene-gotiated with participants. Therefore, in the remainder of this chapter we describe one such attempt at achieving transformation of workplace cultures through reflective inquiry with practitioners on a 'Cancer and Palliative Care Practice Development Programme'.

The Practice Context

The practice context is a large teaching hospital in Northern Ireland, designated as part of the regional Cancer Centre. Medical and surgical cancer specialities exist with outpatient services, general in-patient wards, and an Oncology-Haematology directorate spanning two hospital sites. The number of cancer CNS has increased over this past few years, with most providing a service across the Trust. However, individual post holders have interpreted their roles in various ways according to service demands and previous clinical experience. What appears similar, however, is the tendency to become so engulfed in clinical activity that other aspects of the role are hard to achieve.

Following discussion about this with the palliative care team leader, Liz agreed to facilitate a practice development programme for the CNS with Brendan acting as critical companion (The Cancer and Palliative Care Practice Development Programme). Those invited to participate included: five Macmillan CNS from palliative care, a Macmillan CNS from gynae-oncology, a bone marrow transplant co-ordinator, two CNS for people with lung cancer, and a Macmillan oncology nurse practitioner. Each of the CNS held palliative and or cancer care qualifications, four were educated to Masters level, four had first level specialist practice degrees and two were completing specialist practice courses at the time of the project.

The Development of 'Self' as a Facilitator

The development of facilitators of reflective learning is a key factor in enabling successful reflection to take place. The 'training' of clinical supervisors is something that many organisational strategies focus upon and indeed the importance of training for clinical supervision is recognised in the literature (see, e.g. Wheeler, 2001; Marrow et al., 2002; Bailey, 2004). However, facilitator training is not a one-off activity focusing on achieving a particular set of competencies. Instead, as McGill and Beaty (2001) point out, developing facilitation skills and expertise is a lifelong learning experience.

This lifelong learning approach has been evident in our experience as facilitators and in this section of the chapter we present a reflective narrative exploring Liz's developmental journey as a facilitator with Brendan as her critical companion (Titchen, 2003). This learning journey helped to prepare Liz for the challenges she would face in undertaking the practice development project described in this chapter.

Becoming Aware

A keen interest in developing nursing practice found me (Liz) at the RCN Practice Development week-long residential school. This event marks my 'becoming aware' of the importance of facilitation as a technique to enable learning and where I first recognised its importance in effecting change and development in the workplace. Brendan was the facilitator of the Action Learning Set I was in, and as I watched and listened with an avid interest I observed the skills he used to manage the group, how he paid attention to process, incorporated activities to get us relaxed, and established a climate of learning, where, although we were undoubtedly out of our comfort zones, we felt supported enough to take risks and engage in new ways of learning. One thing that impressed me was the focussed attention he gave to those engaged in communication with him and the positive affect that this had.

Around this time I participated in the RCN Expertise in practice project (Manley et al., 2005), as a Critical Companion to a nurse colleague. Brendan was once again the facilitator involved, acting as Critical Companion to those of us new to the role. This experience deepened my interest in the concept of facilitation. While a formal action learning set structure was not employed, I noted Brendan nonetheless adhered to many of the same processes, such as; investing time in helping us all get to know each other, identifying our expectations of the project, clarifying our values relating to nursing expertise, daily process evaluation and sharing responsibility with us for shaping the programme of work within a participatory framework. Not only were we being valued as 'co-researchers' but I was also impressed that Brendan genuinely seemed to value what I took to be 'ordinary' experience and that he was at pains to ensure such experiential knowledge was made explicit. This I began to realise was the purpose of Critical Companionship (Titchen, 2003; Titchen and McGinley, 2003), at the core of learning from practice and central to the whole notion of practice development. The learning emerging from the project, positive feedback received and Brendan's role modelling of affirmation stimulated a personal and growing desire to develop such facilitation skill and knowledge.

Learning and Doing

Further learning occurred during a two-year clinical leaders' practice development programme that we (our clinical directorate management team) had invited Brendan to develop, lead and facilitate. This time I was a participant as well as an internal facilitator. We engaged in action learning sets twice monthly as well as in various workshops. During this programme I was both 'learning and doing'. The qualities of the facilitator became clearer to me. Brendan's personal interest in individuals and their agendas, his warmth and the equality of attention he gave impressed me. I could see that he worked in an "I: Thou" relationship (Buber, 1984), and although challenge was given, it was always balanced with support. This, along with his receptiveness to high challenge was a refreshingly different way of interacting. I also noted that he did not dismiss contributions or put people down, but tended to use a "yes-and ... ." strategy, where he would acknowledge what was heard and then would offer another perspective, a simple but effective transformational process. Another key learning for me was the way theory was constantly woven into the discussions or workshops but was pitched appropriately to enable relevant learning rather than 'dazzling' us with theory for theory's sake. Flexibility with regards to programme content and consensus decision making seemed to give those of us on the programme a sense of ownership and control. This approach encouraged me, as internal facilitator, to take some initiative and work further with the ward leaders to capture and refine our vision for the clinical directorate and to identify a process for engaging all nursing staff in the development of a shared vision.

Sharing Learning and Taking Risks

Stimulated by the programme I was enthusiastic to share my learning with others, so I set up a co-operative action learning set for colleagues within the Trust who were also interested in practice development. Although we felt 'amateurs' we decided to risk learning by 'doing' action learning and then reflecting on our 'doing' to develop our facilitation skills, an approach consistent with that role modelled on the clinical leaders' practice development programme.

At each step of this journey I was being constantly moved out of my comfort zone, and co-facilitating some workshops with Brendan in coaching mode was no exception. I found these both stressful and difficult and rather than being 'authentic' felt I was acting the part (Rogers, 1983). However, even when I was less than happy with my performance I never felt judged or was made to feel 'stupid'. The value of me as a person was still communicated through relating constantly to me as an equal and helping me to keep things in perspective.

Around this time I had the opportunity to engage in action learning with another UK expert, and began to realise that facilitation styles vary considerably. What I could see as similar was the attention paid to establishing relationship, the focussed attention and the value placed on the person, the skills of questioning, attending and listening, and the importance of process review. What was different was the pace, in terms of increased use of silence, and with less intervention by the facilitator. We were given significant space to muddle through and find our own way. Reflection on this raised my awareness that I was already beginning to favour and echo the style I was accustomed to!

Formalising Learning

By this time I was undertaking an MSc in Advanced Nursing and to gain maximum benefit I shaped my assignments, including a concept analysis, around facilitation. Brendan acted as my dissertation supervisor and through our supervision discussions I felt I was making significant progress in theoretical knowledge. However, it was after a miserable attempt to facilitate an action learning set in front of a leading UK expert that I sat down and undertook a structured critical reflection. Why did I have extreme anxiety when performing in front of facilitators with expertise? Much insight and personal learning resulted from this reflection and subsequent facilitation attempts slowly but steadily improved. I found I understood what I was doing and could draw on appropriate knowledge. This is what Fay (1987) refers to as embodiment, where propositional knowledge is translated into non-propositional knowledge, or put differently from 'know that' to 'know how'.

What really consolidated my learning however, was undertaking the Post Graduate Certificate in Facilitation at the University of Ulster (http://campusone.ulster.ac.uk/) (at the same time as facilitating the Cancer and Palliative Care Practice Development Programme). On this e-learning course, I was both participant and facilitator. I co-facilitated on-line discussion with a number of co-students, as well as participating in critical debate on-line with co-facilitators, in which Brendan again acted as tutor and facilitator, another 'out of comfort zone' experience. The level of debate was much more intense and rigorous than I had experienced heretofore. At first I found this really disquieting, as the discussions on-line would go much wider than the previously agreed topic area. It was after a reflection on this, that I realised I still identified with a 'banking approach' to learning, where chunks of knowledge are cashed out, whereas what we were being encouraged to do was to draw on theoretical and experiential knowledge and integrate it into our practice. Engaging in this type of debate really helped to sharpen my critical thinking ability as did having to produce evidence to benchmark practice against the Royal College of Nursing Facilitation standards (http://www.rcn.org.uk/resources/practicedevelopment/about-pd/processes/facilitation/).

'Self' as Facilitator

It is worth noting that during the course of this learning journey, knowledge of 'self' has increased significantly. My own Christian world view was challenged by the philosophical underpinnings of humanism, existentialism and critical social science. Wider reading and much reflection with respect to this resulted in double loop learning (Argyris, 2002), as I sought to challenge not only my values and beliefs, but how and why I arrived at those values and beliefs. This was an extremely painful process, and if comfort zones had been shifted before, they almost disappeared as I struggled through this disorientating dilemma, eventually emerging with a perspective transformation, through decisive action. It is now with a much deeper understanding and fresh appreciation of the full circle of knowledge imbued in the Christian faith, and of its relevance to me as a facilitator that I rejoice, with love of one's fellow man the foundational ethic. But it was Brendan, as Critical Companion, who helped me to identify how to draw on some of the transformational principles rather than compromising or adopting philosophies or beliefs to which I am opposed. The critical dialogues we engaged in helped to internalise principles that at face value appeared to 'clash' with my espoused Christian values. As Brendan didn't share these Christian values we needed to search for shared meaning in a way that would enable us to transcend particular entrenched positions. We discovered that despite opposing world views, both of us shared a basic respect for persons and a desire to engage with others in a mutually beneficial way to achieve perspective transformation. Thus, consistent with Titchen's critical companionship framework, the learning through this experience was a shared experience and we both developed as facilitators.

This reflective learning account highlights the importance of developing facilitation knowledge, skills and expertise in a systematic way and with the support of a critical companion. The knowledge and skill highlighted in this reflection are consistent with classic theories of facilitation (Rogers, 1983; Heron, 1989) and reflective learning (McGill and Beaty, 2001) and it is these that Liz took to the Cancer and Palliative Care Practice Development Programme described in this chapter. These foundational skills equipped Liz with the confidence to 'go it alone' as a facilitator with the support of a critical companion.

Methodology and Design

The Cancer and Palliative Care Practice Development Programme was located within an emancipatory practice development methodology, as outlined by Manley and McCormack (2003). The aims of the programme were threefold. First, to enable CNS maximise their role potential through a programme of work-based and action learning. Second, to develop the CNS practice development knowledge and skill and third to evaluate the impact of the programme from the perspective of the participants. To determine the effectiveness of the programme in achieving those aims two evaluation questions were agreed:

- How are clinical nurse specialists enabled to maximise their role potential?
- What is the impact of a programme of developmental activities on clinical nurse specialists and their practice?

Conceptual Framework

To link the various components of the programme, a conceptual framework was developed (Figure 5.1). The outer circle of the framework represents emancipatory practice development. Using the tools of critical social science (Fay, 1987), namely *reflection and critique*, it upholds the need to work with *values and beliefs* in a climate of *high challenge with high support* to enable *learning*. Critical social theory also supports the need to conceptualise an alternative *vision* for how things could be which in this case is a vision for the CNS role. It advocates the need to gain new insights and challenge constraining forces within workplace context and culture, which impact both on individuals and on their practice, and demonstrates the necessary leadership to act to bring about change. This depicts the process of enlightenment, empowerment and emancipation outlined by Fay (1987).

Moving inwards, the interconnecting *philosophical principles* circle represents the type of person-centred facilitation used, as well as

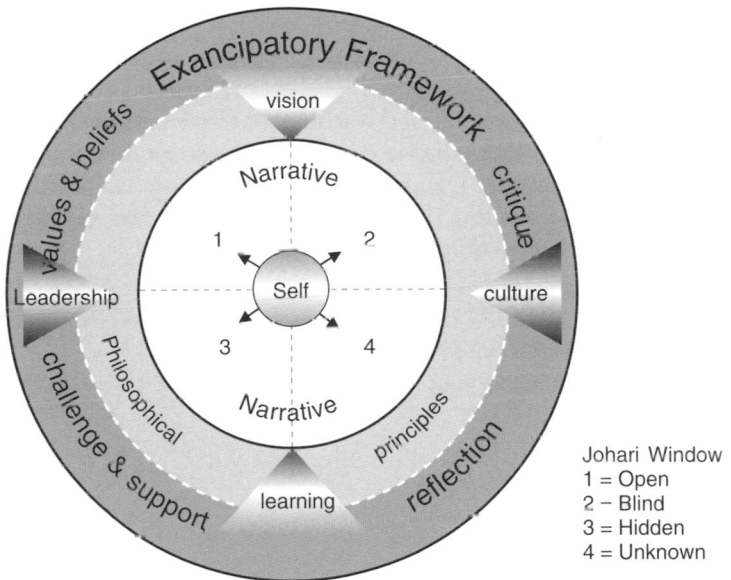

Figure 5.1   Conceptual Framework.

participant experience being the focus of the inquiry. Part of the facilitation role was to enable participants to become aware of possibilities, of making choices and taking responsibility for those choices, in the context of developing their role and their practice. *Narrative* depicted in the pale section is actively used as a way of making sense of experience, by listening to others tell their stories of practice, and through engaging in critical dialogue, new understandings and knowledge emerge. The *four numbered sections* represent Luft's (1970) *Johari Window* feedback and disclosure model, which can be used as a guide to increase personal and interpersonal awareness. The understood aim of the model is to increase the size of the 'open' self, by discovering the 'blind' self (through feedback) and revealing 'hidden' self (through disclosure). The greater the size of the open self, the more effective we are in our relationships with others, and the more effective we are as leaders. Luft (1970) argues that we can get to know ourselves and others better if we take risks in disclosing ourselves and if we hear others' assessment of us. This notion of coming to know *self* better, to know and relate to others has formed a central tenet of the project and provides justification for the various development techniques employed.

Programme of Work

Initially the project was planned to run over one year but with unanimous agreement we decided to continue for a second year. As illustrated in the conceptual framework the programme was structured to enable *learning* around three ongoing action cycles, each beginning with a workshop on the topic.

1. Developing a shared *vision* for the project and the CNS role
2. Understanding the *culture and context* of care
3. Developing *leadership* to effect practice change

We later added an 'emotional intelligence' workshop in response to emerging need, as understanding self in the context of the CNS role became an increasingly significant aspect of the programme. Practice development theory was also woven into the programme, with particular attention to understanding Critical Companionship (Titchen, 2003). The integrated development and data collection methods used are outlined in Table 5.1.

Table 5.1 Integrated Development and Evaluation methods

Activity	Rationale
Reflection on Practice	Use of structured reflection is key to the programme as a means of increasing the size of the 'open' self and is engaged in using various methods such as: • Reflective diaries • Ten minute quick reflections within the group, with verbalised prompts from the facilitator in the form of structured questions, while participants jot down their reflections (kept privately) • Shared structured group reflection on an agreed issue (verbalised) Reflection on action is described by Johns (1996) as a window for practitioners to look inside and know who they are, as they try to make sense of desirable work in their daily practice. Knowing self is an essential prerequisite for knowing and relating to others. Meutzel (1988) argues that the nurse who is self-aware has a special contribution to make in the relationship with patients, and that this self-awareness is essential to practice therapeutically.
Action Learning (AL)	The process of Action Learning (AL) is in itself a means of shared reflection. Action Learning is described by McGill and Beaty (2001) as a facilitated, structured form of group work in which individuals come together regularly over an agreed period of time to learn from each other, with the explicit intention of taking action on the learning. Through the sharing of work-related issues, and utilising strategies of high challenge and support, new insights emerge, which individuals then take responsibility for acting upon.
Values Clarification	Surfacing values and beliefs is a means of heightening awareness of the tension between what is personally espoused and what is enacted in the real world. Such dissonance can be a precursor to action. The methods used ranged from rational questions around beliefs and values (concerning leadership for example), to creative artwork, use of images and poetry.

Continued

Table 5.1 Continued

Creative Arts and Poetry	According to McNiff (1998), creative processes help individuals gain fresh perspectives, access new ways of seeing the world and explore possibilities for action. For example by painting our ideal for the CNS role individually, and then collectively creating a collage from all our ideas, we were accessing hidden parts of our own and others' imaginations and generating a more positive, optimistic climate in which to plan practice change.
Activity Analysis (Disclosure to self)	Activity analysis designed and undertaken by participants, raised their own self-awareness and formed a baseline as to how they operationalized their role. By taking responsibility for this more objective look at how time was spent, and what was being given priority within the role, a more informed debate was had about the need to change.
Role Clarification (Feedback from others)	Within the group a 360° role clarification questionnaire was designed and administered by the CNS thus enabling them to receive feedback from others in relation to how their roles were perceived. This feedback revealed that while the clinical component of CNS work was appreciated there was little understanding of other role components.
Johari Window Proforma	A proforma, based on the Johari Window model, was developed to help the CNS make sense of the collated data from both the activity analysis and the role clarification exercise (Figure 5.3). From this action plans were subsequently formulated. This exercise highlighted the comparison between the current situation and the vision for the role. It is by challenging the contradiction between the realities of every day experience and what is being espoused as the ideal that helps individuals to become enlightened as to their true situation, and may empower them to act to bring about change.
Work-based Learning Objectives	Each participant identified a work-based learning objective to work on. These were areas of practice that they wished to improve, in keeping with adult learning theory as outlined by Jarvis (1983) and Schon (1991).
Care Stories	Identifying the good in everyday practice increasingly became important within the project, hence

Table 5.1 Continued

	the CNS agreed to narrate care stories, as a means of identifying and more fully understanding their own nursing expertise. This exploration of craft knowledge was realised through the application of Critical Companionship facilitation strategies, as illustrated by Binnie and Titchen (2001), with the explicit intention of generating new knowledge from practice. Through story telling, then engaging in critical dialogue, and subsequently undertaking narrative analysis of the taped sessions, the CNS had a raised awareness of their contribution to patient care and the quality of service.
Feedback from Stakeholder Group	An advisory group comprising key stakeholders in the organisation was establishe and through this the feedback obtained helped to inform ongoing development work. This activity enabled the CNS to obtain insight into others' expectations of them with respect to producing tangible project outcomes.

The Developmental Journey

In narrating the group story the first person is used interchangeably with collective nouns as appropriate, to illustrate the processes used and the impact on us all as a group.

A verse of a poem written by Hannah at the commencement of the programme is used in two ways, first to show the type of chaos narrative heard at this time, and second to illustrate our journey of learning.

> Hustle, bustle, noise, clutter, spinning
> Out of control,
> Ideas, goals, plans, but no time to finish
> Does it have to be like this?
> Stop, take stock, think again.

'Hustle, bustle, noise, clutter'

'Chaos' sums up the first few lines of this verse. It is an apt word to describe the messy realities of practice and is referred to by Schon

(1991) as the 'swampy lowlands' of practice. In looking back over the two years we can see how the chaos of the practice setting constantly impacts on us, albeit to varying degrees at different times. Early stories told through action learning clearly illustrated its impact. Presentations described ineffective teamwork, avoidance and denial, medical dominance and avoidance of conflict.

		SELF	
		Known	Not known
Johari Window			
1. *Open*	Known		
2. *Blind*	OTHERS	1	2 *Blind*
3. *Hidden*			
4. *Unknown*			
	Not Known	3	4

We can now see that during those early months the 'blind' Johari windowpane was large within the group. While the impact of practice chaos was keenly felt and vividly described, there was a somewhat resigned despair at the situation, and a sense of it all being subject to powers outside our sphere of control. To reduce the blind quadrant, feedback in the form of high challenge during action learning was given, and concept maps drawn up to give visual impact of the type of disempowered narrative heard. The aim was to enable new insights among the CNS that some action, no matter how small, could be taken to address the situation.

'Ideas, goals, plans'

Line three of the poem can be used to describe the next phase of the project, spanning six months, which were full of *'ideas, goals, and plans'*. The three workshops took place during this time. The first, developing a shared vision for the CNS role, was to help motivate participants to change by conceptualising and verbalising their ideal. From this we agreed on four sub-roles, recognising that education/learning, research and leadership were as important as the clinical component and described our values for each, in terms of what they would look like in practice. At a later evaluation Dolores wrote, 'I found the visioning very challenging, deep down I knew I wasn't meeting all the aspects of the role'.

The next step made explicit the barriers to achieving the vision and the enabling factors to overcome these barriers. Subsequent to this day we designed and undertook an activity analysis and role clarification exercise to check out our assumptions regarding how we spent our time and others' understanding of our role. Overall people understood and valued the CNS clinical input but were less clear about the other sub-roles. In evaluation of this activity Colette said, 'for me using the questionnaire was a huge insight into how others perceive the role'. The activity analysis highlighted various things for individuals but we all agreed the data collection was extremely useful bringing to consciousness how time was spent.

We then had our goal in the form of the vision for the role, and had established the existing state of affairs in relation to how we spent our time and how others viewed the role. The Johari Window proforma enabled us to synthesise this information which helped in identifying steps we could individually take towards maximising our role potential. These we expressed as work-based learning objectives (detailed later in Table 5.2). Workshops exploring culture and leadership were both creative in nature and engendered new insight and learning. In evaluating the impact Bernie said 'These creative days were excellent, considering that no one really wanted to get involved initially and were sceptical, however we now admit how much we all learned about ourselves as individuals and about our organisation'. Themes of action learning sets at this time showed an increased awareness of living up to role expectations and of living up to both one's own and others' expectations. Nine months into the programme we evaluated the progress to date which demonstrated an increasing use of reflective practice with colleagues in the clinical setting (Estelle and Bernie), an example of facilitating others learning through questioning (Gina), role modelling person-centred care (Fiona), and challenging multidisciplinary team colleagues (Colette). In using postcards as a visual image to say where we had got to on the programme Gina described it as, 'crossing the rope-bridge. I'm feeling enthusiastic, I know I still need a lot of courage, I'm still in-between but I'm going to make it over, even then it'll not be over'.

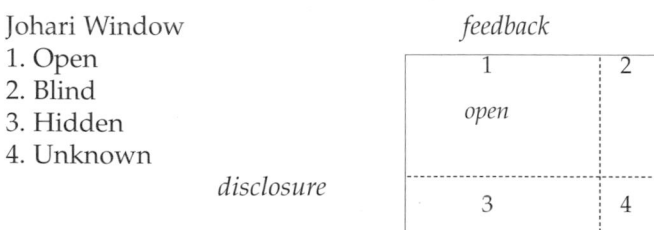

Looking at this period now through the Johari Window we see it as a time when trust within the group was high, feedback and disclosure were significant and we were increasingly 'open' to learning.

But ... does it have to be like this?

'*But*' then came our reality. During the tenth action learning set tension between two group members surfaced. This manifests itself through lack of voice. No one would present an issue; yet, it was apparent that something was going on within the group. As facilitator I chose to challenge this and work with the silence. This provoked anxiety in set members, and some resentment. Gina said 'I think there are issues outside the group that are difficult to bring up here, for fear of causing personal hurt feelings'.

Twice more in close succession group members tried postponing dealing with the issue, the preferred cultural avoidance response resurfacing. Tension in the group was extremely high. Line four of the poem asks '*does it have to be like this?*' I knew if we ignored this emerging problem the growth of the group would be stunted, and what Johns (1992) refers to as 'the harmonious team façade' maintained.

At the height of tension I suggested we stop and do a round of how individuals were feeling, in which emotions were identified as 'sad', 'helpless', 'confused', 'lonely', 'awkward', 'distressed'. Opportunity was afforded for the issue to be addressed, but it became obvious that it was too difficult to speak out even in a safe environment. This silence or passivity is in itself an impoverished way of expression (Belenky et al., 1986). To overcome this hurdle, I suggested we use visual images on postcards to depict our understanding of the situation, as a means of channelling and transforming the emotional energy from a destructive force to a productive exploration. This opened up through metaphor how vulnerable individuals were feeling, that there were interpersonal issues at the route of the problem, and how misunderstandings had escalated into conflict. By drawing on group theory and paying attention to process I was indicating to the group members that they had to take responsibility for themselves and help to negotiate their solutions.

By paying attention to the process I endeavoured to role model dealing with rather than avoiding issues. What we were experiencing was the emotional pain of confrontation. In relation to the Johari Window the 'hidden' was being exposed through the high challenge,

identification of emotions, and metaphorical disclosure of the interpersonal problem.

Johari Window

1. *Open*
2. *Blind*
3. *Hidden*
4. *Unknown*

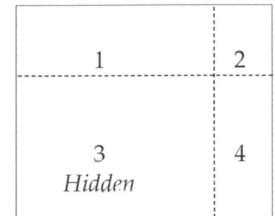

What was unfolding here was in many ways an epitome of situations
encountered by group members in the clinical situation and presented in early action learning sets. The deeply ingrained cultural
norms demonstrated by avoiding confrontation and internalizing
feelings, was a definite pattern. Yet, understanding and handling
those feelings, in the form of emotional intelligence as outlined by
Goleman (1996), is essential for effective interpersonal relationships
and hence for successful teamwork. Facilitating participants to
becoming more emotionally aware was enabled through cathartic
questioning, written reflections on feelings, and 'rounds' as illustrated above. From the group perspective it required high levels of
trust, as in the disclosure there was a risk of being made vulnerable.
A residential workshop on emotional intelligence took place the following month led by an external facilitator. At that, the two set members discovered why they had misunderstandings and engaged with
each other in tentatively exploring it. This was a positive development in the pattern of interaction between team members.

'Spinning out of control'

In January, one year after the programme commenced we presented
our year's work to the advisory panel for the first time. As participants parted some minor tension emerged between set members.
The following month we undertook a shared reflection on the advisory panel's meeting to explore the different perspectives. During
this exercise it became apparent just how diverse those perspectives
were. This all revolved around perceived expectations of the advisory group, predominantly stakeholders from senior management
and multidisciplinary backgrounds, the majority of whom, we perceived, were looking for 'technical' outcomes. We had tried to
explain our learning journey and how we were changing as a result,

but some of us felt this had neither been heard nor understood by a number of the panel members.

Johari Window

1. *Open*
2. *Blind*
3. *Hidden*
4. *Unknown*

1	2
3	4
	Unknown

From a Johari Window perspective the 'open' window was very small, we as a group were 'unknown' to them, as they to us, and we were speaking a practice development language that many of them did not appreciate or understand. During the shared reflection, as facilitator I (Liz) tried to highlight the many political perspectives we needed to be cognizant off and asked, 'why did we have an advisory group?' The response from Angela represented a major challenge:

> you suggested it Liz, ultimately that is the crux of this whole entire experience, we have come to this completely naïve and we have gone along with what has come up as it came up . . . I mean we do this day and daily, but we're just talking about it in a different language now and we've allowed people like [advisory group members] make us feel almost inadequate that we're not doing what . . . do you know what I mean?

As facilitator I was aware of a sinking feeling inside, things seemed to be *'spinning out of control'* but I knew I had to 'hear' her story, even though it was hard to hear. I listened, praised the honesty and attempted to explore the issues with the group, but when another set member who held a different perspective became vulnerable, I interjected by describing a time when I was a participant on another practice development programme. I described the pain of the journey, but also the learning and growth that ensued. My intentions at the time were to provide a holding place amid the pain, and offer hope and encouragement by bringing possibility into view.

'Stop, take stock, think again'

The final line of the poem summarises our position. We had *stopped, we took stock* and offered choice in relation to continuing with the programme. We explored this at some length and everyone opted to stay. We then reconsidered and redefined the purpose of the programme, and identified the enabling and inhibiting factors. We redrafted the ground rules and evaluated the day. Although extremely painful, as a group we felt we had made significant progress. Angela said:

> I liked being able to speak about those issues in a very constructive manner without getting aggressive or angry. I also liked having had the opportunity to be quite open and honest about not only that but other things too and just having the time to take stock really.

To achieve emotional closure we each identified how we were feeling. Angela reported 'I feel relieved and I feel empowered'. What arose as a potential barrier to group survival in terms of high challenge and opposing perspectives became a catalyst for new insights and subsequent growth for us all, through learning about self, others and the organisation. Attention to the process and working collaboratively through honest engagement enabled the transition. However, in thinking with the above story I recognised that by constantly challenging practice and being exposed to others and self-scrutiny, there was real danger of internalising feelings of inadequacy. I could hear the need for what Carl Rogers calls 'prizing' within the group (Rogers, 1983), that is, showing group members that I trusted them, valued them as persons, cared about them, their individual learning journeys and their capacity to flourish. We needed to *'think again'* about the approach taken, and to look for the good.

Making Use of Care Stories

In response to this, at the next learning set, the CNS agreed to recount a clinical situation in which they had made a difference to patient care. After each narration we engaged in critical dialogue to explicate craft knowledge, as outlined in Titchen's (2003) critical companion framework. Attributes of nursing expertise (RCN, 2003), also served as a useful benchmark to our practice. We challenged ourselves by questioning what the added value of clinical nurse specialists might be. This really made us *'think again'* to better understand and re-appreciate our clinical input, and the importance of

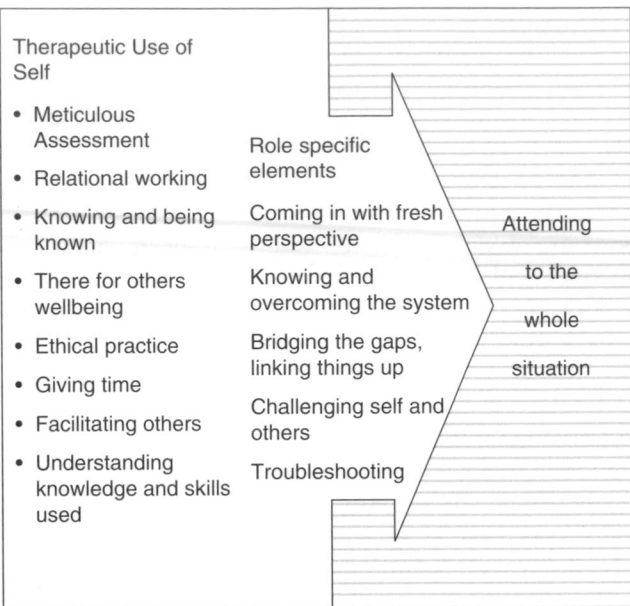

Figure 5.2 Themes from Care Stories.

expressing the small things that make a huge difference to patients. Care stories as inquiry, became a significant feature during the last six months of the programme, with an increasing willingness and critical ability to question our own practice and in so doing release tacit knowledge embedded in our experience. The taped stories as well as the critical dialogue were transcribed verbatim and narrative analysis subsequently undertaken. Key phrases identified in individual stories were grouped to form sub-themes from which overarching themes were agreed (Figure 5.2). These themes will be discussed in more detail later in this chapter.

Evaluating the Impact of the Programme

Towards the end of the two years we spent time reviewing the data and engaging in reflective dialogue to evaluate the overall impact of the programme with respect to the two research questions posed. With reference to the first question, the group story was used to illustrate *how we were enabled to maximise our role potential.* This next section considers *what the impact of the programme was on us and on our practice;* reporting this in terms of project outcomes which, we consider, relate to three main areas.

1. Findings from the care stories
2. Practice development initiatives
3. Increased personal and professional effectiveness

Findings from Care Stories

In listening to each others' care stories we began to appreciate that using self therapeutically is core to our practice and the themes listed under 'therapeutic use of self', although not elaborated on in this chapter, show how in our context we operationalise this. On the other hand, we realise that working in this person-centred way and practising therapeutically is not restricted to Clinical Nurse Specialists. Teasing out the differences between our clinical work as CNS and that of other nurses who may also practice therapeutically became a useful exploration.

The difference emerging from our data is illustrated under the 'Role-specific elements' in the connecting part of the diagram. By virtue of the CNS role we are positioned outside of the clinical setting which at times feels like we are 'out in the ether'. There is a sense in which we then enter situations, but by virtue of that and our experience of cross boundary working, are able to *bring to the situation a fresh or wider perspective.* We *know the system* and how to navigate it. We see the gaps and act to *bridge those gaps, linking* and connecting elements up. We constantly act as a go-between, and find that we need to be prepared to do whatever is required to achieve favourable person-centred outcomes. This often necessitates us *challenging others,* which is *personally challenging* as it requires some risk taking, but with which we persist, for the benefit of the person at the centre of care. We frequently struggle to overcome the hurdles, proactively *troubleshooting* by working with people to help resolve issues. Unpacked in this way each activity can look quite trivial, but when taken as a whole makes a significant statement not only about our contribution but about barriers and weaknesses in the health care context. Finding ways to overcome these and practising in this way necessitates us having personal resilience and a stereoscopic perspective, which culminates in our *'attending to the whole situation'.*

The hidden time commitment in all of this is huge, not only in engaging directly with patients and carers, which we have discovered frequently takes around one and a half hours, but in then going back and forward between internal and external parties to address identified need.

The evaluation of this practice development project was set within a health care trust's organisational context where CNS historically occupy an ambiguous position with little attention paid to anything other than the clinical component of the role. Even with that, we perceived that at times our specific contribution to patient care was poorly understood, hardly surprising as we too had difficulty articulating it. This development programme therefore helped to increase the 'open self' in practice, revealing to us those hidden, taken-for-granted aspects of our work that made a significant contribution to patient care. In listening to our own and each other's stories and by critiquing them new practice knowledge and understanding had emerged. We saw too the importance of acting on this knowledge by rendering these everyday activities visible for others, to enable them become more aware of the contribution CNS can make, not least to the clinical governance agenda. The care stories had identified our effectiveness in minimizing and reducing complaints, and demonstrated that through holistic, personal, interpersonal and system-related interventions, we play a key role in reducing risk and contributing to improvements in the standard of care and quality of service.

Practice Development Initiatives

The impact of the programme on our practice was evidenced through the implementation of work-based learning objectives. These objectives were informed by such things as, individual role clarification exercises, activity analysis, advisory group feedback (which highlighted to us the need to produce tangible outcomes), and the narrative analysis of our care.

In analysing the care stories we realised how much of a facilitation role we actually played, which we had failed to appreciate before, not only with patients and carers, but also within the health care team. In response to this, some of us chose to further develop facilitation skill by constructing it as a personal learning objective, exercised through engaging staff in a parallel process of structured reflection in the ward setting, to help them appreciate their own practice expertise.

Second, in becoming aware that we can offer a 'fresh perspective', one of us opted to draw on this and on a newly found poetic ability, to enable patients to write creatively about their cancer experience. With patients' permission these poems were subsequently projected on screen at the beginning of each multi-professional team meeting, enabling the team to gain 'fresh perspectives' and help set the tone for more person-centred discussion.

A third practice development example associated with the knowledge generated from practice concerned our 'knowing the system' and 'linking things up'. A few of us selected to draw on this knowledge and engaged in patient process mapping and service improvement work as a way of developing the 'links' thus improving the quality of care.

The activity analysis exercise highlighted for some of us how little time we actually devoted to formal education, while action learning sets revealed that any teaching we did do seemed to have little or no lasting impact. In recognition of this, and in learning that emancipatory practice development methodology upholds the need to clarify values and beliefs as a basis on which to build for sustainable practice change, we 'challenged ourselves' to risk working in this new way.

Other tangible outcomes are the production of a staff resource file, an audit of patient waiting times, development of a clinical protocol and the formulation of a research proposal. Table 5.2 summarises these developments in practice and the corresponding component of the CNS role to which they relate.

Increased Personal and Professional Effectiveness

In evaluating the overall worth of the project we took into consideration its impact on us as individuals. Given that Johari Window formed a central tenet of the programme with the explicit intention of enabling us to better know self to know and relate to others, an impact on self knowledge is to be expected. The relevance of this to our roles is evident from the care narrative analysis, with the key theme 'therapeutic use of self'. In addition, 'relational working', 'knowing and being known' and other such themes, illustrate the relevance of fostering self-insight, to become increasingly aware of our own values and prejudices, in order for them not to interfere with the persons for whom we are caring.

From listening to our stories and connecting the narrative threads it is evident that such insight and personal learning has occurred, for example Angela stated, 'I have become more aware of who I am and what I am'. Estelle, in looking back reflexively, can see self as changed, 'I am a totally different person in lots of ways'. However, there is no sense in us feeling we have arrived, as Dolores put it 'I have been enabled to look at self in a reflective / critical manner and see the blind spots and then work on at increasing awareness of self / behaviours in situations'. The themes of learning and personal development associated with reflection and a resulting increase in self-confidence in dealing with difficult issues dominate the data. Johns (1998) suggests that without critical reflection to better know self, a nurse's personal way of knowing will not inform theory nor bring about transformative change and subsequent improvement in practice.

From a practice development perspective McCormack and Wright (2000) affirm there can be pain associated with transformative work, because to change can be costly both personally and professionally and argue that significant support is required. This project echoes those findings. While there is an increased sense of responsibility for leading and enabling others to develop their practice, the ability to achieve this amidst the 'chaos' of an increasingly complex workplace context with its constant clinical pressure remains extremely challenging. It would be misleading and naïve to suggest that we have completely altered how we operationalize our role, rather there is evidence of small role changes. For Bernie the change is in 'starting to say no . . . recognising that not all things are as important'. The following evaluation by Angela seems to sum up the thinking within the group.

> The programme has allowed us the opportunity to really explore the components and look at where we want to be, and look at what the vision is, and help us work out a way, enable us to approach it in a way that we might try to spread ourselves out throughout those components a bit more evenly. Listening this morning it's evident people have blossomed in their role. I've been one of the big cynics but I do feel that there has been some blossoming. We have evidence we are now working in the different components a little bit more effectively.

In summary therefore our collective evaluation reveals:

- Increased personal insight, growth and development
- Ability to interact better with others

Table 5.2 Summary of Developments in Practice

Participant	Developments in practice outcomes	CNS Role Component
Individual participants	• (a)Enabling patient through the expression medium of poetry. (b) Use of patient poetry to develop a more person-centred ethos at the multi-disciplinary team meeting.	Clinical Leadership
	• Contribution to patient pathway mapping	Leadership
	• Use of structured reflection with ward staff	Education / learning
	• Development of protocols for reviewing patients at a nurse-led clinic for use by others	Leadership & Education
	• Facilitating a clinical leader to improve communication among the multi-professional team using a practice development approach	Leadership
Small group of participants	• Production of a resource pack for staff	Education / learning
	• Taking a lead in patient pathway mapping	Leadership
	• Audit of patient waiting times	Leadership
	• Mapping availability of patient information	Leadership
	• Development of a research proposal into carer and user experience of the service in negotiation with a charitable organisation	Research
Larger group of participants	• Facilitating learning in various wards throughout the Trust in relation to particular clinical issues. Rather than 'teach', the CNS applied practice development learning gained on the programme to work with staff's values and believes, to enable new insights.	Education / learning

- An increased ability to reflect and to question our practice
- Increased ability to think laterally
- Enhanced focus
- Greater appreciation of our own skill and knowledge
- Increased self-confidence

Conclusion

This chapter has argued for the development of frameworks that facilitate systematic process of inquiry, within a learning climate of high challenge and high support. Clinical supervision offers one such approach, but we have also illustrated how through the use of developmental processes (rather than a particular model), we have systematically engaged in transforming practice culture through learning to understand 'self'. The conceptual framework used in the study described, illustrates how the use of a heuristic device such as the Johari Window assisted in connecting the various elements of the programme, focusing on 'what is hidden' about self and others, thus becoming more open to learning to increase personal effectiveness.

Accessing everyday experience is complex and we should never underestimate the challenges associated with doing this work. However, although it is difficult and complex, it doesn't require 'magic' (e.g. control, prediction and extraction) but instead it requires a commitment to a rigorous and systematic understanding of everyday experience. We know that effective workplace cultures value staff as 'persons' and therefore it is essential that opportunities are created for staff to have the space to actually stop amid the complexity and chaos of practice, and to take the time to look back at practice and the cultures in which practice happens. Practitioners can learn how to shape workplace cultures and come to know how they are shaped by those cultures. Establishing mechanisms for systematically developing, narrating and analysing shared practice stories can be an enlightening process in its own right and can add much to our understanding of the processes used and the outcomes experienced. The CNS development programme presented in this chapter was labour intensive and expensive in terms of facilitator's and participants' time as compared with many clinical supervision projects which are often smaller in scale. However, the evidence from this sustained and systematically developed programme of work speaks for itself and perhaps challenges us to think about 'programmes' of clinical supervision rather than stand-alone small-scale projects.

The final word goes to Hannah (a participant on the programme described here) who, in a creative reflection, captures the essence of the importance of structures and processes that enable growth of 'self' through reflection:

> Uncertainty, apprehension, confusion,
> What's it all about?
> 'Reflection', 'emancipation', 'transformation', what does it mean?
> 'High challenge? high support?' – frightening!
>
> Light begins to filter through,
> Flicker by flicker, glimmer by glimmer,
> Openness, trust, warmth,
> Painful moments, leading to growth
> Understanding, knowledge and change.

References

Argyris C (2002) Double-loop learning, Teaching, and Research, *Academy of Management Learning and Education*, 1(2): 206–218.

Argyris C (1999) *On organisational learning*. Blackwell Business, Massachusetts.

Argyris C and Schon DA (1989) *Theory in Practice: Increasing Professional Effectiveness*. Jossey-Bass Publishers, London.

Bailey C (2004) Supervision. Reflecting on training courses – the heart of the matter. *Counselling and Psychotherapy Journal*, 15(10): 36.

Belenky M, Clinchy B, Goldberger N and Tarule J (1986) *Women's Ways of Knowing*. Basic Books, New York.

Benner P, Tanner C and Chesla C (1996) *Expertise in Nursing Practice: Caring, Clinical Judgement and Ethics*. Springer Publishing Company, New York.

Binnie A and Titchen A (2001) *Freedom to Practise: The Development of Patient-Centred Nursing*. Butterworth Heinemann, Oxford.

Buber M (1984) *I and Thou*. Prentice Hall, New Jersey.

Fay B (1987) *Critical Social Science*. Polity Press, Oxford.

Freshwater D (2000) Crosscurrents: against cultural narration in nursing. *Journal of Advanced Nursing*, 32(2): 481–484.

Goleman D (1996) *Emotional Intelligence*. Bloomsbury, London.

Heron J (1989) *The Facilitators' Handbook*. Kogan Page, London.

Jackson D, Clare J and Mannix J (2002) Who would want to be a nurse? Violence in the workplace – a factor in recruitment and retention. *Journal of Nursing Management*, 10(1): 13–20.

Jarvis P (1983) *Professional Education*. Croom Helm, London.

Johns C (1992) Ownership and the harmonious team: barriers to developing the therapeutic nursing team in primary nursing. *Journal of Clinical Nursing*, 1: 89–94.

Johns C (1996) Visualising and realising caring in practice through guided reflection. *Journal of Advanced Nursing*, 24: 1135–1143.

Johns C and Hardy H (1998) In: Johns C, Freshwater D (eds) *Transforming Nursing Through Reflective Practice*. Blackwell Publishing, Oxford.

Kitson A, Ahmed LB, Harvey G, Seers K and Thompson DRF (1996) From research to practice: one organisational model for promoting research-based practice. *Journal of Advanced Nursing*, 23(3): 430–440.

Luft J (1970) 2nd edition, *Group Processes: An Introduction to Group Dynamics*. Mayfield Publishing Co., California.

Manley K, Hardy S, Titchen A, Garbett R and McCormack B (2005) *Changing Patients' Worlds Through Nursing Practice Expertise:* Royal College of Nursing, London.

Manley K (2004) Transformational culture: A culture of effectiveness. In: B McCormack, R Garbett and K Manley (eds) *Practice Development in Nursing*. Blackwell Publishing Ltd, Oxford.

Manley K (2000) Organisational culture and consultant nurse outcomes: Part 1 organisational culture. *Nursing Standard*, 14(36): 34–38.

Manley K and McCormack B (2003) Practice development: purpose, methodology, facilitation and evaluation. *Nursing in Critical Care*, 8(1): 22–29.

McCormack B (2004) Person-centredness in gerontological nursing: an overview of the literature. *International Journal of Older People Nursing (in association with the Journal of Clinical Nursing)* 13(3A): 31–38.

McCormack B and Titchen A (2001) Patient-centred practice: an emerging focus for nursing expertise. In: Higgs J and Titchen (eds) *A Practice Knowledge and Expertise in the Health Professions*, pp. 96–101. Butterworth-Heinemann, Oxford.

McCormack B and Wright J (2000) Achieving dignified care for older people through practice development. *Nursing Times Research*, 4: 340–352.

Muetzel P (1988) Therapeutic nursing. In: Pearson A (ed.) *Primary Nursing: Nursing in the Burford and Oxford Nursing Development Unit*. Croom Helm, London.

Marrow CE, Hollyoake K, Hamer D and Kenrick C (2002) Clinical supervision using video-conferencing technology: a reflective account. *Journal of Nursing Management*, 10(5): 275–282.

McKenna BG, Smith NA, Poole SJ and Coverdale JH (2003) Horizontal violence: experiences of Registered Nurses in their first year of practice. *Journal of Advanced Nursing*, 42(1): 90–96.

McGill I and Beaty L (2001) *Action Learning*. Kogan Page, London.

McNiff S (1998) *Trust the Process: An Artist's Guide to Letting Go.* Shambhala, London.

Royal College of Nursing (RCN) (2003) *Expertise in Practice Project*: Final Report. RCN, London.

Rogers C (1983) *Freedom to Learn for the 80's.* Merrill, Ohio.

Schon DA (1991) *The Reflective Practitioner: How Professionals Think in Action.* Aldershot, Avebury.

Titchen A (2003) Critical Companionship: part 1. *Nursing Standard*, 18(9): 33–40.

Titchen A and McGinley M (2003) Facilitating practitioner research through critical companionship. *NT Research*, 8(2): 115–131.

Titchen A and Higgs J (2001) Towards professional artistry and creativity in practice. In J Higgs and A Titchen (eds.) *Professional Practice in Health, Education and the Creative Arts*, pp. 273–290, Blackwell Science, Oxford.

Wheeler S (2001) Supervision. Are supervisors born or trained? *Counselling and Psychotherapy Journal* 12(10): 28–29.

Wilson V, McCormack B and Ives G (2005) Understanding the workplace culture of a special care nursery. *Journal of Advanced Nursing*, 50 (1), 27–38.

Winter R and Munn-Giddings C (2001) Action research as an approach to inquiry and development. In: R Winter and C Munn-Giddings (eds) *A Handbook of Action Research in Health and Social Care*, pp 9–26, Routledge, London.

Johari Window Proforma

Known   not known
self

1. Open   known | 1 | 2 |
2. Blind   others
3. Hidden   not known | 3 | 4 |
4. Unknown

Johari Window (Luft, 1970)

The Activity Analysis represents 'what I see I do' (Disclosure to myself)

The Role Clarification is 'what others see me do' (Feedback from others)

Clinical Practice

What does the activity analysis say about me in my role in relation to clinical practice?
What do others (role clarification) say about me in relation to clinical practice?

1. What do I know about my clinical practice that others also know?
2. What do they see about my role that I do not see?
3. What do I Know that I do in my role that they do not see?

Education and Learning

What does the activity analysis say about me in my role in relation to education and learning?
What do others (role clarification) say about me in relation to education and learning?

1. What do I know about my role in education and learning that others also know?
2. What do they see about my role in relation to education and learning that I do not see?
3. What educational things do I know that I do in my role that they do not see?

Leadership

What does the activity analysis say about me in my role in relation to clinical leadership?
What do others (role clarification) say about me in relation to clinical leadership?

1. What do I know about my clinical leadership that others also know?
2. What do they see about my clinical leadership role that I do not see?
3. What do I know that I do in relation to clinical leadership that they do not see?

Research

What does the activity analysis say about me in my role in relation to research?
What do others (role clarification) say about me in relation to research?

1. What do I know about my contribution to research that others also know?
2. What do they see about my role in relation to research that I do not see?
3. What do I know **that** I do in my role in relation to research that they do not see?

Figure 5.3 Johari Window Proforma.

6

Literature Review: Clinical Supervision Evaluation Studies

Veronica Bishop

SYNOPSIS

While much has been written of the potential of clinical supervision to improve patient care and to develop professional growth of practitioners since its formal introduction to nursing in the 1990s, much of the 'evidence' to support this potential is anecdotal. With varying degrees of success, attempts have been made to evaluate its effectiveness and in this chapter I have attempted to bring together some of those studies that have been subjected to peer review. For many the most important issue about clinical supervision is its impact on clinical practice. In this chapter, I have highlighted how research is trying to grapple with this – and it is encouraging that there are indicators to build on for those who are willing to be hard-nosed in their support!

Introduction: Fashion and Feasibility.

Butterworth noted (1998; p. 186):

> it appears fashionable to make no progress on any new development unless they can somehow be tied to patient-led outcomes and evidence based practice, as though these laudable aims were achievable overnight.

Of course it is reasonable – particularly with high demand and limited resources to meet those demands – that today's health care culture requires evidence to support any intervention, particularly one that is costly in terms of time, expertise and therefore, money. However, the complexity of human interactions cannot be so easily quantified. For example, in asking the single question 'is clinical supervision effective' three central issues are raised. Effective for whom? The patient, the practitioner, the employing organisation? While we have established in previous chapters that clinical supervision is about helping practitioners to reach their optimum in terms of clinical competence and confidence, how do we measure its success? Many aspects of nursing, particularly the creation of a therapeutic environment, are difficult to isolate, and as Fowler and Dooher noted (2001), it is a false assumption that lack of measurability indicates lack of usefulness. Conversely, it is equally misleading to assume that practices that are difficult to measure are in any way on a higher intellectual plane.

The impact within the United Kingdom of policy initiatives, supported by professional leaders (these are discussed fully in Chapter 1) resulted in a flurry of activity around clinical developments and practices, one of which was that a questionnaire survey was sent to 1221 practising nurses, midwives and health visitors in England to identify the characteristics of optimum practice (Butterworth and Bishop, 1995). Clinical supervision was identified as one of the 18 key requirements for optimum practice. As one respondent in the study stated:

> Patient care is only as good as the nurse who provides it. Good patient care comes from a nurse who is motivated, has the relevant knowledge, is willing to question and change her practice as required ... ' (p. 31)

Interestingly, another participant, identified by her senior manager as an expert mentioned her surprise at being selected stating

> I'm surprised that I've been nominated as an expert, no one has ever bothered to tell me before' (p. 30)

I have selected these two quotes as they encompass two key elements of clinical supervision, those of reflective practice and support. This very large sample of practitioners endorsed the value of clinical supervision, which they identified as one of the key requirements for optimum practice, seeing its value as embracing a supportive environment for clinical activity and personal development. Since that survey was carried out the vocabulary may have changed a little, and 'clinical competence' be used instead of 'optimum practice', but the underpinning concepts do not change. This endorsement of clinical supervision was supported by the work of Bowles and Young (1999) who found that participants engaged in clinical supervision in their study were willing to examine and change practice, a view earlier noted by Tingle (1995) and more recently by Lipp and Osborne (2000). Scanlon and Weir (1997) found that all participants felt very positively about clinical supervision, as it made them feel valued, certainly a response that I have obtained when speaking to recipients of supervision. In a small study by Bishop and Freshwater (2000), the data clearly indicated that sessions enabled focus on practice and shared learning, and facilitated improved coping mechanisms. The professional support gained on a personal level, and the opportunity to consider personal development was appreciated and an overall view voiced that the quality of care given was *perceived* to have improved since receiving clinical supervision. Overall scores from the Manchester Clinical Supervision Scale (Winstanley, 2000) indicated a positive response to clinical supervision and its effective delivery. The one negative factor in this study was the difficulty respondents had in finding time for sessions – a complaint recurring in many studies.

Finding the Right Tools

The report 'The New NHS – Modern and Dependable' (DoH, 1998) stated that trusts

> should encourage a self-evaluative and responsive nature amongst ... nurses that will allow clinical practice to evolve and reflect emerging evidence of effectiveness.

Winstanley (2001; p. 211) holds the view, and I concur, that:

> Now that clinical supervision has an established role to play in the working practices of the nursing workforce, effective evaluation of clinical supervision is one of the most important challenges which currently face nursing.

To evaluate anything some kind of measurement has to be taken of selected aspects or indices. In clinical supervision there are currently no established standards to guide the researcher, and as a consequence different studies use different outcomes in attempts to establish its effectiveness. This in itself need not be problematic, and as long as consistency is used throughout the study the results can be valid. However, it does preclude any aggregation of data, thus depriving an interested community of consistent data from which to inform and develop policy. There is one exception to this, the work of Winstanley, using the Manchester Clinical Supervision Scale (MCSS) derived from a multi-site study in the UK (Butterworth et al., 1997), will be discussed later in this chapter.

Carson stressed (1998; p. 163) the need to develop measures to evaluate clinical supervision that is based on the principles of reliability, validity and utility. He also acknowledged the role of qualitative methods, particularly in illustrating the 'lived experience'. The examples of evaluative studies that are highlighted in this chapter demonstrate the developing body of knowledge on clinical supervision, from its implementation, application and reception, to its relationship to clinical outcomes. The somewhat national bias owes to the fact that literature searches indicate that the different English speaking educational programmes in North America (mainly at Masters level), and the varied connotations of the word 'supervision' offer little relevant evaluative material published from across the Atlantic. Yegdich noted that despite numerous well-attended conferences where clinical supervision was the sole topic, it remains to be seen how idiosyncratically Australians will forge clinical supervision in their own image (Yegdich, 2001; p. 264). She went on to insist that clinical supervision is essential for the therapeutic use of self in nurse–patients interactions. However, work has been undertaken in Scandinavia, particularly in Sweden (Severinsson and Hallberg, 1996) and in Finland where clinical supervision started in the 1950s, but moved at a slow pace (Paunonem and Hyrkas, 2001). In the 1980s, an extensive Ministerial survey in Finland revealed that the need for clinical supervision far outweighed its supply. Subsequent work focused on a model of integrated clinical supervision with education and training, and is moving towards collaboration where evaluation research will provide new perspectives for clinical supervision and international collaboration (Hyrkas et al., 2003). Besides translation, an instrument developed and tested in another culture requires systematic validation and this study focused on the translation process of the MCSS for testing in Finland, work carried out collaboratively between the Universities of Tampere and Manchester. Results indicated that clinical supervision emerged as the main

- Defining and agreeing ground rules
- Devising and monitoring implementation plans
- Provision of training for all parties
- Developing and monitoring a list of supervisors
- Selecting indices for evaluation

Figure 6.1 Setting the scene for evaluation.

concept in a learning environment, suggesting that the concept of clinical supervision is taking firm root beyond the United Kingdom (Saariksoki and Leino-Kilpi, 2002).

The first step towards developing consistent, comparable data that could be aggregated in evaluating clinical supervision in nursing and health visiting was discussed in a review paper (Butterworth et al., 1996) stemming from the flood of activity around clinical supervision in the United Kingdom at that time. This review recognized the necessity of establishing sophisticated tools that would provide health care providers with evidence that the time, money and effort of clinical supervision were resources well spent. In identifying some evaluation techniques to assist practitioners and managers to assess the utility and usefulness and impact of clinical supervision the items in Figure 6.1 were considered important.

The last of these items is the tricky bit and the suggested audit trail at the time was through sickness rates, staff satisfaction scales, patient complaints, recruitment and retention and critical incident maps.

The Manchester Clinical Supervision Scale (Winstanley, 2000)

In the absence of any validated specific instrument for the task of measuring the effectiveness of clinical supervision the Manchester study (Butterworth et al., 1997) used five selected instruments that had been validated in other work settings. These were considered to be sensitive to the normative, formative and supportive elements of the Proctor model of supervision, which was most commonly used nationally. These were:

- The Minnesota Job Satisfaction Scale (Weiss, 1967)
- The Maslach Burnout Inventory (Maslach and Jackson, 1986)

- The General Health Questionnaire (Goldberg and Williams, 1988)
- The Nurse Stress Index (Harris, 1989)
- Cooper Coping Skills (Cooper et al., 1988)

Information gained from the project was vast, with 586 nurses involved in the study, and it is from the refinement of these data, and from a series of retesting and revalidating in further studies that the current MCSS is derived. It is the first validated assessment instrument designed specifically for the evaluation of the effectiveness of clinical supervision, and the copyright holder considers that data from this scale can inform and be a part of systems of clinical governance (Winstanley, 2001; p. 222).

It's Good to Talk?

Hill (1989) a community psychiatric nurse, provided what was possibly the first review of the literature around clinical supervision, and while encouraged by its apparent usefulness concluded that there was little evidence from the literature of any real debate on the subject in the nursing profession. In a later substantive review of publications from various specialities Butterworth and Faugier (1992) came to a similar conclusion, although they identified that some progress was to be found in psychiatric nursing and health visiting literature. Proving the truth of this Sloan, a nurse specialist in cognitive and behavioural psychotherapy, published a review that focused on perceived good characteristics of supervision from the supervisees' perspective (Sloan, 1998). His particular interest was promoted by the earlier work of Fowler (1995), and focused on the perceptions of nurses of the elements of good supervision (a key area discussed fully by Freshwater in chapter 4.). Sloan concluded that while earlier studies began to illuminate a complex aspect of the supervisory relationship, a 'variety of methodological limitations have constrained their findings (p. 2). In 1999, Gilmore was commissioned by the United Kingdom Central Council for Nursing (UKCC) to carry out a review of evaluative work on clinical supervision and found that the minimal amount of work in this area precluded a balanced assessment of the impact of clinical supervision in the United Kingdom. The same could not be said now, although the difficulty of equating clinical supervision with good nursing care remains difficult.

Notwithstanding this challenge Sloan has continued valuable work to investigate fundamental process issues in clinical supervision and their influences on nursing outcomes (Sloan, 1999, 2000; Sloan and Watson, 2001). Later, building on the seminal work by Butterworth et al., (1997) and the refinement of that work by Winstanley (2000) Edwards et al. (2005) sought to identify, from a sample population of mental health nurses in Wales, those factors that impact upon the success of clinical supervision, building on earlier work in the Principality (Edwards et al., 2003). They found that clinical supervision evaluated more positively where sessions lasted over an hour and were held at least on a monthly basis. Perceived quality was also higher where supervisors had been chosen rather than designated, and where sessions took place away from the workplace. The authors noted the need for organisational and cultural change for successful implementation of clinical supervision, a comment made by most researchers in this field.

Clinical Outcomes: The Challenge

The identification of indices of clinical effectiveness or positive clinical outcomes is dependent on the type of patient–nurse interaction prescribed. For example, in mental health settings nurses' or therapists' interactions are focused largely around their therapeutic relationship with the patient. Clinical supervision therefore needs to focus on what they bring to that relationship. The 'healing' relationship that is inherent in general nursing requires the nurse or therapist to identify problems from which interventions can be determined. Individual indices matched to individualised patient care are most likely to provide 'hard' evidence of effective clinical supervision, but could evolve into a tick box mechanistic exercise that may not necessarily mean that the nurse is engaging in reflective practice and developing the use of self to maximise a therapeutic environment.

To date most of the published work to evaluate clinical supervision has focused on the perceptions of practitioners alone, examples of which are cited above. As Cottrell (2001) noted, conceptual and methodological problems make it very difficult to attribute any change in a client's health status to an individual practitioner's clinical supervision. The study by Hallberg and Norberg (1993) had suffered this dilemma. Despite finding that the intervention of clinical supervision assisted nurses in their responses to demented patients, particularly where the burden of care was great, they were unable to reveal whether or not the patients' experience was improved. Braving the inherent problems of measuring the clinical efficacy of clinical supervision, Green (1999) used a utilisation-focused evaluation as a flexible framework, guided by the work of Patton (1986) on which to evaluate a programme of clinical supervision in one NHS trust. The majority of participants had been using the framework as part of their reflective practice within clinical supervision sessions and had an awareness of the processes involved in change. Importantly, they were familiar with the use of Critical Incident Analyses, where clinical issues are identified and some attempt is made to assess underlying errors, causes and contributory factors. One of the requirements of the study was evidence of how clinical supervision had positively influenced practice, and all but one of the interviewees were able to describe such a situation. Kemppainen (2000) also utilised the critical incident technique to identify what evidence practitioners could provide that demonstrated changes in practice. Much more work needs to be done in this area if clinical supervision is to offer 'hard currency' at the cost-effectiveness counter. However, the need to help practitioners to develop their motivation for providing quality approaches to practice – motives that may have brought them into their chosen profession in the first place (as noted by McCormack and Henderson in Chapter 6) but have often been lost in the organisational systems of work – must not be overlooked or discounted. Improved patient care, as Cottrell (2000) comments, depends on the provision of time for reflection on practice as a trust's commitment to an organisationally endorsed process.

Leadership and Supervision

> Nursing is not recognised for the leaders it produces. Rather, leadership – the ability to lead, guide, direct or show the way – is a quality often lacking in the nursing profession. (Marriner, 1994)

Nursing is the bedrock of health care, and when I speak of nursing I am talking about qualified people who bring knowledge and experience to the patient – whether through direct contact or at the board table. Nurse leadership, particularly in the United Kingdom has,

I suspect, never been as clear as we longer serving members of the profession like to think (Bishop, 2004), this despite the suggestion that nursing has a great need of clinical leaders to produce climates for creativity on a mass scale in all areas of nursing (Salvage, 1990). Johns (2003) contends that clinical leadership is the cornerstone for innovation and development, citing successive government documents that set a background for innovation and change, with strong nursing leadership. However, although devolution has brought interesting changes in health care and evidence of professional coherence in Scotland, Northern Ireland and Wales (Greer, 2004), the allegiance in England with management has, in the view of many, served the nursing profession badly. Greer observed that England has carried the most visible experiments in health policy with its market-based agenda, and he commented on the restlessness and often heedlessness of English policy. This lack of cohesion and often opportunistic approach to health care has had a profound effect on nurse leadership in England, and there is a view that the nursing profession has never been more vulnerable as it is at present. Reasserting the raison d'etre of nursing – focusing on its clinical function – is not to take a step back into Nightingale and the Crimea! It is about empowerment.

> Clinical supervision is only one strategy by which to empower nurses, but it could be a very potent and supportive one.

Where historically nurse leaders in the United Kingdom rose in the main through the ranks of the now abolished regions, and with the gradual integration of senior nurses at trust level into the management framework, the opportunity for professional peer review and collegiate support has been severely eroded. Clinical supervision, properly implemented can meet some of these essential professional needs. Nursing lacks the coherence of other care disciplines – its positive strength in being fluid and responsive can too easily become a source of professional destruction. Now we seem to be caught in a web of strong threads that stem from such sources as gender stereotyping, medical dominance, political game playing, resource deprivation and inadequate professional leadership at many levels (Marriner, 1994; Freshwater et al., 2002; Collinson, 2002) which conspire to keep us in the place where others would have us. Nurses have a poor record of supporting each other, another reason why we have provided an easy target for those seeking to marginalise us. It is time for us to take stock, to promote and support our articulate and strategic thinkers, and to let them shine. Hargrove (1998) argued that the leaders of today and the foreseeable future need to have collaborative attitudes and knowledge-creating skills, and the ability to empower others – very much in contrast with the traditional hierarchical model to which nursing across the world is accustomed, but totally in keeping with the concepts of clinical supervision. The studies highlighted in this next section focus particularly on leadership skills within the context of clinical supervision. Further material which will be useful to the reader linked to this may be found in chapter 5 on the supervisory process.

Severinsson and Hallberg (1996) studied the clinical supervisors' views of their leadership role in the supervisory process, and the personal qualities and styles. Analysis revealed two specific approaches to supervision; the emotional connection and the cognitive supervisory style. Supervisors' personal qualities indicated a willingness to show understanding – in particular bringing out genuine feelings and confirmation with their supervisees. Their views of their leadership role showed that high values were given to three factors; techniques in providing clinical supervision, responsibility for facilitating the process and creating a climate conducive to supervision, and the ability to focus on the main themes. Freshwater et al. (2001) used a multi-method approach that would generate the depth and richness of data required to evaluate the implementation of clinical supervision in the nursing staff of a prison service in the United Kingdom. Utilising the broad methodological and philosophical framework of action research, and drawing on elements of ethnography and reflexivity (Rolfe, 1998; Freshwater and Rolfe, 2000), this study focused particularly on the development of leadership skills through clinical supervision and reflective practice, and found that while clinical supervision, to be effective, must be owned by staff, it is most likely to occur where an advocate for clinical supervision was identified. The authors noted that while this advocate was not necessarily a senior staff member, they were people who demonstrated leadership skills and were able to overcome many of the real and perceived barriers to the implementation of clinical supervision. This reflects other studies where leadership skills appear to determine the success of any planned change

(Butterworth, 1998; Bishop and Freshwater, 2000) Johns (2003) also linked the concept of clinical leadership with clinical supervision, and evaluated a project that aimed to facilitate growth of leadership through supervision. He found that the organisational culture was less than sympathetic and that those participating were generally willing but unable to significantly develop their leadership ability. He suggested that while working with practitioners through clinical supervision was undoubtedly a powerful way of working towards enabling them to realise desirable practice, aspiring to radical change may be a stage too far within an existing culture.

Clinical Supervision: Stress Reducer?

In the United Kingdom there is a substantial body of evidence to suggest that NHS staff suffer high levels of stress (Payne and Firth-Cozens, 1987; Anderson et al., 1996; Weinberg and Creed, 2000). Health care staff are working under increasing amounts of pressure, and have to balance growing levels of stress from increased workloads, constant changes in management structures and policy directives against the dissonance from lowered standards due to limited resources in terms of staff and care materials. Benner and Wrubel (1989) identified a number of reasons why nursing is stressful, not least the huge personal and emotional demands of the work, and the lack of professional acknowledgement by a mainly male-dominated organisation. Johns (1995) also acknowledged that organisations regarded nurses' contribution to be inferior to that of doctors, and Farrington (1995) outlined how stress is depressing, demoralising and de-motivating for nurses. The fact that nursing in England and Wales has a 12 per cent turnover rate with high recruitment problems and with 28 per cent of nurses claiming to find their working conditions stressful (Workforce survey for nurses, midwives and health visitors, 2004) is surely an indicator that some constructive measure needs to be introduced to support nurses in their work.

In the 1995 major multi-site clinical supervision study 18 English and 5 Scottish sites were investigated. Using the component elements of clinical supervision suggested by Proctor (see Chapter 2), those being the normative, restorative and formative components the first step of the evaluation study was to investigate the effectiveness of staff support. The results of this study are published in detail elsewhere and shortcomings in the instruments utilised are

- Reduction in sick leave
- Raised job satisfaction
- Improved recruitment
- Improved retention
- Reduced stress

Figure 6.2   Some indices studied.

acknowledged (Butterworth et al., 1997). Further data were obtained through in-depth interviews (White et al., 1998) and taken into account when later evaluative measures were designed. However, overall the study indicated that participants who had not had clinical supervision were more emotionally exhausted than those in the groups receiving clinical supervision, and that those who did eventually receive it showed symptoms of stress to be reduced. Cottrell (2000) used the Pressure Management Indicator (Williams and Cooper, 1998) to examine stress levels in a group of community nursing staff, followed by stress management interventions including the introduction of clinical supervision. While the author was cautious as to the generalisabilty of his findings, clinical supervision was shown to be effective as helping to reduce occupational stress, despite the confusion arising from differences in definition. More recently Hill (2004) carried out a study, based on earlier work by Butterworth et al. (1996), that involved speech and language therapists, hospital-based occupational therapists, dieticians and physiotherapists in a Midlands area. Some of the indices that were studied are shown in Figure 6.2.

Overall the evaluation indicated that burnout related to depersonalisation was reduced, and feelings of personal accomplishment were raised with a positive impact on professional development and skills.

Shared Learning, Shared Goals

Clinical supervision has always played an important part in therapists' professional practice but there is a dearth of literature on how this should be done (Hill, 2004). To combat this Hill established a non-managerial clinical supervision learning programme that involved speech and language therapists, hospital-based occupational therapists, dieticians and physiotherapists. The benefits of training and shared understanding of what is being implemented are clear in this report, something that was missing when I carried out a survey in the early days of UK implementation (Bishop, 1986). In this survey I sent a questionnaire to all the trust nurses executives in England and Scotland, except for the 23 sites involved at that time in the Department of Health study (Butterworth et al., 1997). My aim was to find out what activity, as opposed to superficial interest, was ongoing around clinical supervision. While the data indicated a great deal of activity, there was a marked lack of preparation and support for those involved, which undoubtedly will have accounted for the subsequent reduction in participants across the country, as indicated in the Kings College study (2005) discussed below. Farrington (1995) and Kohner (1994) have all noted that advanced education is needed for such a sophisticated concept, as does Scanlon (1998) who is emphatic stating that:

> It must be understood that clinical supervision requires clearly planned intervention by skilled practitioners with advanced training in individual, group and organisation dynamics. (p. 150)

Scanlon goes on to outline contextual issues surrounding clinical supervision and its application to nursing practice, emphasising the need for grounded theory and for advanced education and training within the context of higher education. Much of this view appears to meet with agreement in Northern Ireland, where the Nursing and Midwifery Advisory Group have drawn up best practice guidelines for mental health nurses having clinical supervision (DHSSPS, 2003). These guidelines underline the importance of training for all concerned. Clinical supervision is seen as central to the successful introduction of clinical and social care governance, and seen as fundamental to the development of safe and effective practice. The evaluation of effective training packages is an obvious next step for policy makers with an eye for quality care and reflective, supported practitioners.

Perhaps the largest study carried out on clinical supervision is that by Davey et al. (2006) which reports on the experiences of 1918 diplomate nurses in their early career, 18 months after qualification from the adult, child, learning disability and mental health branches, based on the elements formative, supportive and normative of the Proctor model (see Chapter 2). The study design employed a panel survey in which a nationally drawn cohort of diploma course qualifiers was sent a series of questionnaires at regular intervals from qualification onwards (Marsland and Murrells, 2000). As clinical supervision was just one aspect of a study that explored nurses' career pathways and aspirations the number of questions that could be included in the questionnaire about clinical supervision was restricted. Findings showed that just over half the learning disability and mental health diplomates were receiving clinical supervision compared with approximately one third of those graduating from the adult and child branches. While the majority of nurses questioned considered that their needs were met in terms of assistance with setting learning objectives, and discussing incidents that occurred at work, over a quarter of supervisees in each branch wanted more discussion of such incidents.

> Of particular concern is that many wanted more supervision in relation to new clinical skills, professional practice and with reflection on practice. (Davey et al., 2006)

There was also substantial unmet need in terms of evaluation of their performance and constructive feedback about their clinical skills. Encouragingly, there was little unmet need in all branches for discussing relationships with staff or for discussing relationships with patients. Emotional support, the restorative aspect, was where there was most unmet need, particularly in mental health, although the majority felt they were given sufficient emotional support in supervision, with nurses in the adult branch least likely to want more emotional support.

Evidence from the data in this chapter suggest that clinical supervision as a supportive mechanism for nursing staff in carrying out their work is worthy of very serious consideration. One wonders if we will soon reach the stage where an employer's responsibility in these areas will be clearly mandated.

Conclusion

In this chapter, I have highlighted studies that have sought to evaluate various components of clinical supervision, with particular emphasis on stress reduction, shared goals and clinical leadership, and clinical outcomes. The Manchester Clinical Supervision Scale is discussed, and its potential to impact on clinical governance. It is apparent from this review that the key to any successful implementation of clinical supervision is the need for a cultural change, not only within employing organisations, but also in the mindset of health care professionals. There is a need for practitioners to acknowledge their centrality in patient welfare and embrace continuous shared learning and skill acquisition.

References

Anderson WRJ, Cooper CL and Willmott M (1996). Sources of stress in the NHS. A comparison of seven occupational groups. *Work and Stress*, 10(1): 88–95.

Benner P and Wrubel J (1989) *The Primacy of Caring: Stress and Coping in Health and Illness*. Addison-Wesley, Wokingham.

Bishop V and Freshwater D (2004) Looking ahead: the future for nursing research. In: Freshwater D and Bishop V (eds) *Nursing Research in Context. Appreciation, Application and Professional Development*, p. 196, Palgrave Macmillan, Basingstoke.

Bishop V and Freshwater D (2000) Clinical supervision: Examples and pointers for good practice. Report for University of Leicester Hospitals Education Consortium.

Bishop V (2004). Editorial. *Nursing Times Research*, 9(2): 164–165.

Bowles N and Young C (1999) An evaluation study of clinical supervision based on Proctor's three function interactive model. *Journal of Advanced Nursing*, 30(4).

Butterworth A. (1998). The potential of clinical supervision for nurses, midwives and health visitors. In: Bishop V (ed.) 1st ed. *Clinical Supervision, Some Questions, Answers and Guidelines*. MacMillan/NTResearch, Basingstoke.

Butterworth T and Faugier J (1992) *Clinical Supervision and Mentorship in Nursing*. Chapman and Hall, London.

Butterworth T and Bishop V (1995) Identifying the characteristics of optimum practice: findings from a survey of practice experts in nursing, midwifery and health visiting. *Journal of Advanced Nursing*, 22: 24–32.

Butterworth T, Bishop V and Carson J (1996) First steps towards evaluating clinical supervision in nursing and health visiting. 1. Theory, policy and practice development. A review. *Journal of Clinical Nursing*, 5: 127–132.

Butterworth T and Bishop V (1995) Identifying the characteristics of optimum practice: findings from a survey of practice experts in nursing, midwifery and health visiting. *Journal of Advanced Nursing*, 22: 24–32.

Butterworth T, Carson J, White E, Jeacock J, Clements A and Bishop V (1997) *It's Good to Talk: An Evaluative Study in England and Scotland*. Manchester University, Manchester.

Carson J (1998). Instruments for evaluating clinical supervision. In: Bishop V (ed.) *Clinical Supervision in Practice. Some Questions, Answers and Guidelines*. MacMillan/NTResearch, Basingstoke.

Collinson G (2002) The primacy of purpose and the leadership of nursing. NTResearch, 7(6): 403–411.

Cooper C, Sloan J and Williams S (1988) *Occupational Stress Indicator Management Guide*. NFER-Nelson, Windsor.

Cottrell S (2001) Occupational stress and job satisfaction in mental health nursing: Focussed interventions via evidence based assessment. *Journal of Psychiatric and Mental Health Nursing*, 8(2): 157–164.

Davey B, Desousa C, Robinson S and Murrells T (2006) The policy-practice divide: who has clinical supervision in nursing? In press. *Journal of Research in Nursing*, Sage Publications, London.

Department of Health and Social SPS (2003) Clinical supervision for mental health nurses in Northern Ireland: Best practice guidelines. DHSSPS.

Department of Health (1998) The New NHS – Modern and Dependable. DoH, London.

Edwards D, Cooper L, Burnard P, Hannigan B, Jugessur T and Fothergill A (2003) The effectiveness of clinical supervision for community mental health nurses. School of Nursing and Midwifery, University of Wales, Cardiff.

Edwards D, Cooper L, Burnard P, Hanningan B, Adams J, Fothergill A and Coyle D (2005) Factors influencing the effectiveness of clinical supervision. *Journal of Psychiatric and Mental Health Nursing*, 12(4): 405–414.

Farrington A (1995) Models of clinical supervision. *British Journal of Nursing*, 4(15): 876–880.

Fowler J (1995) Nurses' perceptions of the elements of good supervision. *Nursing Times*, 91(22): 33–37.

Fowler J and Dooher J (2001) Clinical supervision in multi-disciplinary groups. In: Cutliffe J, Butterworth T, Proctor B (eds) *Fundamental Themes in Clinical Supervision*. Routledge, London.

Freshwater D, Walsh L and Storey L (2001) Developing leadership through clinical supervision. *Nursing Management*, 8(8): 10–13.

Freshwater D, Walsh L and Storey L (2002) Developing leadership through clinical supervision in prison healthcare. *Nursing Management*, 8(9): 16–20.

Freshwater D and Rolfe G (2000) Critical reflexivity: a politically and ethically engaged research method for nursing. *NTResearch*, 6(1): 526–538.

Freshwater D, Walsh L and Storey L (2001) Prison health care: Developing leadership through clinical supervision. *Nursing Management*, 8(8): 10–13.

Gilmore A (1999) Review of the United Kingdom evaluative literature on clinical supervision in nursing and health visiting. UKCC, London.

Goldberg D and Williams P (1988) *Users' Guide to the General Health Questionnaire*. NFER-Nelson.

Green AJ (1999) A utilisation focused evaluation of a clinical supervision programme for nurses and health visitors in one NHS trust. *Journal of Vocational Education*, 51: 494–504.

Greer S (2004) Four Way Bet: How devolution has led to four different models for the NHS. The Constitution Unit, London.

Hallberg IR and Norberg A (1993) Strain among nurses and their emotional reactions during one year of systematic clinical supervision combined with the implementation of individualised care in dementia nursing. *Journal of Advanced Nursing*, 18: 1860–1875.

Hargrove R (1998) *Mastering the Art of Creative Collaboration*. McGraw Hill, New York.

Harris P (1989) The Nurse stress index. *Work and Stress*, 3(4): 335–336.

Hill J (1989) Supervision in the caring professions: a literature review. *Community Psychiatric Nursing Journal*, 9(5): 9–15.

Hill J (2004) The non-managerial clinical supervision learning programme. Evaluation report. West Midlands.

Hyrkas K, Appelquvist-Schmidlechner K and Paunonen-Ilmonen M (2003) Translating and validating the Finnish version of the Manchester Clinical Supervision Scale. *Scandinavian Journal of Caring Sciences*, 17(4): 358.

Johns C (1995) The value of reflective practice for nursing. *Journal of Clinical Nursing*, 4: 23–30.

Johns C (2003) Clinical supervision as a model for clinical leadership. *Journal of Nursing Management*, 11(1): 25–34.

Kemppainen J (2000) The critical incident technique and nursing care quality research. *Journal of Advanced Nursing*, 32: 1264–1271.

Kohner N (1994) *Clinical Supervision in Practice*. Kings Fund Centre, London.

Lipp A and Osborne P (2000) Clinical supervision and clinical governance: the art and science of bridge building. *Journal of Clinical Excellence*, 2: 3–8.

Marriner AC (1994) Theories of leadership. In: Hein CE and Nicholson MJ (eds) *Contemporary Leadership Behaviour* (4th ed) Lippincott Company, Philadelphia.

Marsland L and Murrells T (2000) Sampling for a longitudinal study of the careers of nurses qualifying from the English pre-registration Project 2000 diploma course. *Journal of Advanced Nursing*, 31 (4): 953–943.

Maslach C and Jackson S (1986) *The Maslach Burnout Inventory*. Consulting Psychologist Press, Palo Alto, CA.

Patton MQ (1986) *Utilization –Focused Evaluation*. 2nd ed. Sage, London.

Paunonem M and Hydkas K (2001) Clinical supervision in Finland – history, education, research and theory. In: Cutliffe J, Butterworth T, Proctor B (eds) *Fundamental Themes in Clinical Supervision*. Routledge, London.

Payne R and Frith Cozens J (1987) *Stress in Health Professionals*. Chichester, Wiley.

Rolfe G (1998) The theory practice gap in nursing: from research-based practice to practitioner based research. *Journal of Advanced Nursing*, 28(3): 670–672.

Rounds LR (2001) A North American perspective on clinical supervision. In: Cutliffe J, Butterworth T, Proctor B (eds) *Fundamental Themes in Clinical Supervision*. Routledge, London.

Saarikoski M and Leino-Kilpi H (2002) The clinical learning environment and supervision by staff nurses: developing the instrument. *International Journal of Nursing Studies*, 39: 259–267.

Salvage J (1990) The theory and practice of the 'New Nursing'. *Nursing Times*, 86(4): 42–45.

Scanlon C (1998) Towards effective training of clinical supervisors. In: Bishop V (ed.) *Clinical Supervision in Practice: Some Questions, Answers and Guidelines*. 1st.ed. MacMillan/NTResearch, Basingstoke.

Scanlon C & Weir WS (1997) Learning from practice? Mental health nurses' perceptions and experience of clinical supervision. *Journal of Advanced Nursing*, 26: 295–303.

Severinsson EI and Hallberg IR (1996) Clinical supervisors' views of their leadership role in the clinical supervision process within nursing care. *Journal of Advanced Nursing*, 24(1): 151–161.

Sloan G (1999) Good characteristics of a clinical supervisor: a community mental health perspective. *Journal of Advanced Nursing*, 30: 1713–1722.

Sloan G (2000) The supervisory relationship: are we forgetting something? Netlink: *The Psychiatric Nursing Research Network*, 14: 7–8.

Sloan G and Watson H (2001) Illuminative evaluation: evaluating clinical supervision on its performance rather than the applause. *Journal of Advanced Nursing*, 35 (5): 664–673.

Sloan G (1998) Clinical supervision: characteristics of a good supervisor. *Nursing Standard*, 12 (40): 42–46.

Tingle J (1995) Clinical supervision is an effective risk management tool. British Journal of Nursing, 4: 794–796.

Weinberg AM and Creed F (2000) Stress and Psychiatric disorder in health-care professionals and hospital staff. *The Lancet*, 355, Feb 12th.

Weiss DJ (1967) Manual for the Minnesota Satisfaction Questionnaire. Minneapolis, MN. Industrial Relations Centre, University of Minnesota.

White E, Butterworth T, Bishop V, Carson J, Jeacock J and Clements A (1998) Clinical supervision, insider reports of a private world. *Journal of Advanced Nursing*, 28(1): 85–92.

Williams S and Cooper CL (1998) Measuring occupational stress: Development of the pressure management indicator. *Journal of Occupational Psychology*, 3(4): 306–321.

Winstanley J (2000) Manchester Supervision Scale. *Nursing Standard*, 14(19): 31–32.

Winstanley J (2001) Developing methods for evaluating clinical supervision. In: Cutliffe JR, Butterworth T, Proctor B (eds) *Fundamental Themes in Clinical Supervision*. Routledge, London.

Yegdich T (2001) An Australian perspective on clinical supervision. In: Cutliffe J, Butterworth T, Proctor B (eds) *Fundamental Themes in Clinical Supervision*. Routledge, London.

7

Instruments for Evaluating Clinical Supervision

Jerome Carson

SYNOPSIS

Considerable progress has been made in evaluating clinical supervision since the last issue of this book. Nurses may be surprised to note that research into clinical supervision with nurses, exceeds research conducted with other professional groups on the same subject. In this chapter, I again stress the need to develop measures to evaluate clinical supervision that are based on the key psychometric principles of reliability, validity and utility. The Manchester Clinical Supervision Scale is described in depth, and the findings from independent research with this scale are reported. Data from the Special Hospitals' Nursing Staff Stress Survey are presented which illustrate the importance of clinical supervision on stress process measures. There is still much we do not know. Qualitative methods are important, though often under-utilised, especially in illustrating the so-called lived experience of clinical supervision. The impact that good clinical supervision has on patient outcomes is one that tantalisingly remains out of reach.

Introduction

> Research in supervision is the biggest joke in our profession. There is no distinct body of knowledge to uncover. (Holloway, 1995; p. xi)

Supervision is an assumed rather than proven educational benefit. There are plenty of published articles of a theoretical or anecdotal nature, but precious few that have conducted any empirical investigation of the supervision process and its outcomes. (Green, 1995; p. 41)

Despite its role in serving as the foundation for our training and practice, surprisingly little is known about clinical supervision from an empirical standpoint, (Milne and James, 2005; p. 6)

The first quotation is taken from the field of counselling and the second and third from clinical psychology. All three might equally well be drawn from the field of nursing. It is a myth that clinical supervision (CS) per se is a helpful process. There are good supervisors and bad supervisors. It seems likely that how supervisees perceive their supervisors will have a strong impact on how they feel about supervision and how it impacts both on them and also on the care they provide for their patients.

Clinical Supervision in Nursing

The UKCC in a position statement on clinical supervision (UKCC, 1996), stated that *'Evaluation of clinical supervision is needed to assess how it influences care, practice standards and the service. Evaluation systems should be evaluated locally'* (Key statement 6). The statement went on to make the point made earlier, that there is a lack of information on the benefits and outcomes of CS. More recently, CS has been central in meeting the requirements of clinical governance. This is the framework whereby NHS Trusts are accountable for their services and for promoting adequate care standards (DOH, 2000). Simms (1993), stated that *'there is a growing and acknowledged awareness of and commitment to the value of supervision and the supervisor relationship,'* yet she too was forced into the conclusion that there was little published research. Faugier (1996; p. 53) commented, *'Until recently little of any substance had been published in the nursing literature, and the absence of empirical data on clinical supervision remains widespread in all fields, particularly nursing.'* As I suggested earlier, this last statement is now contradicted by a number of good studies conducted in the nursing field.

A typical early study conducted on CS is that published by Ritter et al. (1996). In this paper, Susan Ritter and her colleagues described the supervision framework that they developed for general nursing students undertaking clinical experience in psychiatric wards. They gave helpful detail about the methods they utilised with students, such as critical incident analysis, life charts and genograms (the last are a type of family tree that illustrate the relationship between the patient and the rest of his/her family, also showing at a glance which members may have died). However, they provided no information on how students perceived these experiences. Other questions remain unanswered. Is their method better than previous methods? What aspects of the supervisory process are most beneficial for students? So while they helpfully inform us about what methods they used, there are no data on the evaluation of these methods.

Equally, Faugier (1996) provided a helpful model of the key requirements of positive supervisory experiences. She suggested that supervisors needed to be generous, rewarding, open, willing to learn, thoughtful and thought provoking, humane, sensitive, uncompromising in standards, adaptable and practice focused, to provide a safe relationship and to establish trust. Apart from providing an example of the model in action (Butterworth and Faugier, 1992), there is no evidence to support this model, despite its intrinsically appealing nature.

The Proctor model of CS (Proctor, 1986; Proctor and Inskipp, 2001), has been one of the most influential models in the field. Proctor conceived of supervision as fulfilling three main functions. She referred to these as normative, formative and restorative. The normative or managerial aspect of supervision implies an element of overseeing or monitoring standards. This involves caseload management, making the supervisee aware of organisational policies and procedures and checking record keeping. Within our own mental health service, computerised record keeping means that any employee can examine the case records of any patient! Butterworth (1996) suggested that the normative element could be evaluated by audits of clinical supervision through looking at sickness and absence rates and by surveys of staff satisfaction. The restorative or supportive aspects of clinical supervision are concerned with the creation of a supervisory relationship in which the employee feels valued and understood. It involves a recognition of the stressors inherent in the nursing role. In my own professional work as a clinical psychologist, it is now considered good practice to inform clinical psychology trainees that the job is inherently stressful and this needs to be addressed in CS. The restorative or supportive element can be measured by scales such as the Maslach Burnout Inventory (Maslach and Jackson, 1986). This scale looks at elements such as the degree to which nurses are emotionally drained by their work (see below for a fuller description). This has some similarity to the recently articulated concept of emotional labour (Mann and Cowburn, 2005). The third and final element is the formative or educational component. This is concerned with the identification and development of skills in supervisees and the integration of theory with practice. Butterworth (1996) suggested a number of ways in which the formative element could be evaluated. He recommended Trust wide educational audits to check that staff are still involving themselves in continuing education. He also mentions the use of audio and video tape to enable supervisors to monitor the development of supervisees' therapeutic skills. One of my own trainees recently insisted that I listen to a tape of one of his sessions with a client. I was amazed to discover how structured and systematic he was in the session. Fortunately, this tallied with my own assessment of his abilities, so it was not as great a shock as it might have been!

Approaches to Evaluating Clinical Supervision

The simple use of quantitative measures to evaluate the complex process of CS is no guarantee of reliability or validity. During my own training as a clinical psychologist from 1981 to 1984, all trainees were rated at the end of each placement on a number of key competencies, such as report writing. The rating scale used had a number of categories. These were, 'Excellent', 'Very good', 'Better than average', 'Average', 'Below average' and 'Fail'. An analysis of these ratings by the Regional Tutor Anne Richardson, showed that almost 90 per cent of trainees were at least better than average!

It is interesting to look at contemporary practice. I mainly supervise trainees at the Institute of Psychiatry. At the middle and end of each placement I have to rate the trainee on thirty-one different dimensions. Each dimension is rated as 'needs attention', 'satisfactory', 'good' or 'not applicable'. The scale covers a range of competencies that trainees are expected to demonstrate during their six month placements. These cover dimensions such as, 'choice of assessment methods', 'implementing appropriate methods of evaluations of interventions', 'understanding relevant ethical issues', 'appreciating the inherent power imbalances between practitioners and clients and how abuses can be minimised', 'using supervision to reflect on practice, and making appropriate use of feedback', and the like. In turn the supervisee rates the supervisor on thirteen dimensions.

These cover issues such as 'supervisor style- availability, approach-
ability', 'clinical advice- appropriate to level, flexible, alternative
approaches', 'support- help around challenging cases, difficulties
with colleagues'. Trainees now have more scope to comment on
supervision. A previous assessment of supervisors only had four
rating categories. In addition, the supervisor rates the trainees'
strengths and needs. The supervisee is also able to comment on their
own ratings. The reliability of an assessment such as this is open to
question. It is the ultimate tick box assessment. Virtually all ratings
are either satisfactory or good!

Perhaps in the light of such experiences the largest clinical
psychology training course at University College London moved
towards a qualitative form of assessment. Their form assessed
fourteen specific competencies such as 'professional behaviour',
'relationship with colleagues', and 'interviewing skills'. Supervisees
are also able to rate their supervisors on the quality of their supervision. While this is more of a qualitative approach to supervision, it
may be better at capturing the dynamic nature of the supervisory
process. Speaking as a supervisor who has completed both types of
assessment, a combination of both methods seems preferable. For
instance Surrey University, asks for a rating on each dimension on a
four-point scale and then asks the supervisor for specific instances of
the behaviour in action. For example, in response to a question on
knowledge of diversity, I was able to state that a trainee had completed a number of directed reading assignments, had gone for a
seminar with a colleague who was the Trust lead in this field and
had also worked with a range of clients from diverse backgrounds
during his placement.

Mechanisms for evaluating student and supervisor performance
are carefully worked out. In contrast, the supervision of qualified
staff leaves much to be desired. At best, a short record may be provided of what has been covered in sessions, but there is never any
rating of the quality of the supervisory process!

Principles Guiding the Selection of Measures to Evaluate Clinical Supervision

In terms of a quantitative evaluation of CS, the approach of Streiner
(1993a) was helpful. Streiner provided a checklist for evaluating the

content of rating scales. This checklist can be applied to scales that are used to evaluate CS. The following issues are critical.

(A)   Item Analysis

1.   Item selection. How are items selected for scales? In most instances, items are taken from previous scales. Streiner commented, *'Borrowing from one source is plagiarism, but taking from two or more is research!'* (Streiner, p. 141). Clinical observation, expert opinion, patients' reports or theory may also provide items for scales.
2.   Item analysis. Once selected for inclusion, items then need to be subjected to detailed item analysis. This looks at issues such as endorsement frequency, restrictions in the range of responses and comprehension. The main reason for developing any questionnaire is to be able to discriminate between groups of people who complete it (Golombok and Rust, 1989).
3.   Item discrimination analysis. Items need to be included that best discriminate between high and low scorers on the dimensions being measured.
4.   Item–item and item total correlations. Correlations range from +1.0 to −1.0. The first suggests that two variables are strongly associated, the latter that they are not. If items do not correlate at a level of greater than 0.2 with the total score on a dimension, they may be measuring something completely different. Equally, if items correlate too highly with each other, there may be an element of item redundancy. These points are illustrated by Brown et al. (1995).

(B)   Reliability

In essence, reliability refers to the accuracy or precision of a measure. If we have a scale that assesses anxiety, its reliability is to do with how accurately it measures anxiety. This can be assessed in a variety of ways. *Internal consistency* is concerned with how consistently the individual scores on items assessing the same phenomenon. If there are ten questions that assess anxiety, we can compare the individual's scores on the first five items versus their scores on the second five (split-half reliability). Alternatively, we could compare their scores on odd-numbered items, 1,3,5,7,9 against their scores for even items 2,4,6,8,10 (odd–even reliability). The most widely used method for assessing internal reliability is Cronbach's alpha (Cronbach, 1951). Modern computer-based statistical-based packages such as SPSS (Norussis, 1993; Kinnear and Gray, 1994; Foster, 1998), make the process of estimating scale reliability a fairly straightforward business. A second type of reliability is *test–retest reliability*. If we administer our anxiety scale to individuals on two occasions a week apart, there should be a high correlation between their scores on both occasions, unless there have been major changes in their lives in between. A third type of reliability is called *inter-rater reliability*. This last form of reliability is important with behaviour rating scales. For instance using the Health of the Nation Outcome Scale (HoNOS), do two raters give similar ratings on the same patient? We can assess this by showing the raters a patient on video and having them make ratings of the patient's problems. This can be evaluated as percent exact agreement, though there are most sophisticated measures such as Cohen's weighted kappa.

(C) Validity

The validity of any scale is based on whether it measures what it purports to measure. Rather like reliability, it is assessed in a variety of ways. *Face validity* asks the deceptively simple question, on the face of it, do the items look as if they are measuring what they are meant to? *Content validity* takes this a step forward. It asks, does the scale measure the most relevant elements of the construct being examined? For instance, a scale of depression needs to cover both biological aspects of depression, such as weight loss, sleep disturbance, diurnal variation, loss of libido and so on, with psychological aspects such as pessimism, hopelessness, helplessness and guilt and the like. *Criterion validity* comprises both concurrent and predictive validity. Concurrent correlational validity assesses the degree to which scores on a scale correlate with existing measures of the same phenomenon. For instance, how do Beck Depression Inventory scores correlate with scores on the Hospital Anxiety and Depression Scale or the Centre for Epidemiological Depression Scale. Predictive validity is when a person's score on a scale is used to make predictions about his or her future behaviour. For example, staff scoring high on a measure of occupational stressors might be more likely to have higher sickness absence rates than staff with low occupational stressor scores. Finally, *construct validity* is to do with the accumulation of research evidence that is built up over time with respect to a particular construct. Eysenck (1980) conducted a whole range of studies that linked the phenomena of extroversion and introversion with biological factors such as conditionability. The issue of conditionability is tested through a series of learning theory paradigms, for example, eye blink conditioning. Here a light may be shone before a puff of air is squirted into the eye. After a number of pairings of the light and the air puff, the former is presented on its own. The conditioning response is then tested. Eysenck has shown that criminals do not condition easily and suggested that this was why they did not learn moral codes and laws so well. Extroversion can be reliably assessed using the 90-item Eysenck Personality Questionnaire (Eysenck and Eysenck, 1975).

In considering the issues of reliability and validity, the researcher needs to know which specific populations that these dimensions have been tested on. It used to be said that psychology was the study of the American undergraduate. The reason for this was that American students had to participate in experiments to earn course credits. Consequently, a large number of questionnaires were standardised with undergraduate populations. These would not therefore be representative of the population at large. Clinical scales need to be developed with established clinical populations.

(D)   Utility

The final issue to consider is utility. How long does it take to complete a measure? How much training is needed to administer, score and interpret the scores? Equally important is how accessible the scale is, how much does it cost to purchase and is there a manual? The above description has necessarily been brief and has omitted more complex issues such as factor analysis, which are central to the notion of test construction. Readers who wish to learn more about scale construction should refer to Streiner and Norman (1989). Streiner has also written a number of user-friendly accounts of other aspects of research methodology in a series of papers in the Canadian *Journal of Psychiatry* (see Streiner, 1990, 1993b, 1994, 1995, 1996a,b, 2002a,b,c; Goering and Streiner, 1996).

The Manchester Clinical Supervision Scale

The problems of evaluating CS were manifested in the influential Clinical Supervision Evaluation Project (Butterworth et al., 1997).

This project tried to evaluate the core components of CS as articulated by Proctor (1986). The normative element was assessed by the Minnesota Job Satisfaction Scale (Weiss et al., 1967). Restorative elements were measured by the Maslach Burnout Inventory (Maslach and Jackson, 1986), the General Health Questionnaire (Goldberg and Williams, 1988), the Nurse Stress Index (Harris, 1989) and the Cooper Coping Skills Subscale (Cooper et al., 1988). Of these standardised rating scales, only the Minnesota Job Satisfaction Scale and the Maslach Burnout Inventory were found to be sensitive to changes brought about through participation in CS. The biggest gap in the project was the lack of a scale to assess the effectiveness of the supervision received by participants. This gap was filled later by the development of the Manchester Clinical Supervision Scale (MCSS) (Winstanley, 2000; Winstanley and White, 2003).

The strength of the MCSS is that it assesses all three elements of the Proctor supervision model. The scale was developed out of the Clinical Supervision Evaluation Project. Items for the new scale were drawn partly from the questionnaire responses from the study, and also from individual interviews conducted by the study researchers (White et al., 1998). The original scale comprised fifty-nine questions. This was piloted in five centres with a range of nursing specialisms included. Staff were asked to rate statements about the CS they received on a five-point scale from strongly agree to strongly disagree. Factor analysis was then used to establish an underlying structure for the scale and to reduce the number of items to forty five. A second study of 467 nurses was then conducted, again from five UK centres. A further factor analysis on these data resulted in a 36-item scale.

The MCSS has seven factors. The first, 'Trust/Rapport' (seven items), is linked to the normative or restorative element, for example, '*I can unload during my CS session*'. The second, 'Supervisor Advice/Support' (six items), is linked to the restorative function, for example, '*My supervisor gives me support and encouragement*'. The third, 'Improved Care or Skills' (seven items), is linked to the formative function, for example, '*CS improves the quality of care I give to patients/clients*'. The fourth, 'The Importance Value of CS' (six items), is linked to the normative function, for example, '*CS is unnecessary for experienced/established staff*' (reverse scored). The fifth, 'Finding Time' (four items), links to normative or restorative functions, for example, '*It is important to make time for CS sessions*'. The sixth, 'Personal Issues' (three items), is tied to restorative elements, for example, '*I feel less stressed after seeing my supervisor*'. Finally the last, 'Reflection' (three items), is linked to the formative function, for example, '*CS sessions facilitate reflective practice*'.

Winstanley and White (2003) report the MCSS is sensitive at detecting high and low scorers. Internal consistency within and between subscales is high on Cronbach's alpha. Test–retest reliability for the subscales and total score are all above 0.9. The scale cannot however be used as a before and after measure, as it can only be completed when an individual has experienced CS. A high score on any of the subscales is said to reflect a high degree of effectiveness of the CS received. A high overall scale score is said to reflect effective CS.

Independent Studies that have Used the Manchester Clinical Supervision Scale

1. Edwards et al. (2005)

In carrying out the All-Wales Community Mental Health Nursing Stress Survey (Burnard et al., 2000), the researchers were surprised that CS was not identified as a way of coping with work-related stress. They speculated that this might be either as Community Psychiatric Nurses (CPNs) may not have been offered CS or alternatively that the CS on offer was of poor quality. They decided to carry out a study to look at what factors impacted on the effectiveness of CS with community mental health nurses. The study used the MCSS along with a demographic questionnaire. This asked about issues to do with the length and frequency of supervision sessions, whether CPNs could choose their supervisors and whether supervision was individual or group in format. Of the 817 CPNs surveyed, completed questionnaires were received from 260, representing a 32 per cent response rate. Of these 210 had experience of CS, reflecting a 26 per cent response rate from the total sample. The main findings were as follows:

- Longer sessions led to more effective ratings of supervision. The mean score for CS sessions less than 45 minutes was 133.94 but 142.90 for sessions lasting longer than an hour.
- More frequent supervision was also associated with higher ratings. The mean score for a frequency of less than monthly sessions was 141.54. Supervisees who only had supervision on a quarterly basis had a score of 124.14.

- Being able to choose your own supervisor was associated with higher supervision ratings, 142.36 versus 131.32. Supervisees who chose their own supervisor also had significantly higher scores on the Trust/Rapport and Supervisor Advice/Support subscales.
- While the majority of respondents received supervision within their own workplace, 158 vs 22, CS was more effective when conducted off-site, 147.14 versus 136.99. Reflection, Trust/ Rapport and Improved Care or Skills were also rated higher when CS was conducted off-site.
- There were no differences in effectiveness of CS between individual or group formats.

Edwards and colleagues conclude that time, space, choice are important elements for effective supervision and that short infrequent CS is of limited value.

2. Hyrkäs (2005)

Hyrkäs (2005) conducted a large Finnish study of 569 nurses drawn from a wide range of health care organisations throughout Finland. The researcher used the MCSS, the Maslach Burnout Inventory, the Minnesota Job Satisfaction Scale as well as a demographic questionnaire. The main findings from this study were:

- Female staff rated supervision as more effective, 143.6 versus 136.0.
- Younger staff rated supervision as less effective than other staff, 138.7 for staff younger than 30, but 144.0 for staff in the 41 to 50 age group.
- Acting as a supervisor yourself, increased your ratings of your own supervision 146.4 versus 140.5.
- Choosing your own supervisor was associated with higher MCSS ratings, 144.0 versus 134.9.
- More frequent supervision was rated higher. Weekly supervision was 144.3, versus 140.8 for infrequent supervision.
- Group supervision was rated as less effective than individual supervision, 136.5 versus 145.0. This was however related to the size of the supervision groups, with bigger groups being associated with lower ratings.

The presentation of findings of effective supervision and burnout and job satisfaction is somewhat complex. I have attempted to simplify these below. If staff are divided into a group that perceives supervision as being highly effective and a group that perceives CS as being ineffective, then the following findings emerge with respect to burnout. Staff in receipt of ineffective CS are more likely to suffer from high depersonalisation burnout, 8.2 per cent versus 4.2 per cent, and low personal accomplishment 6.8 per cent versus 1.8 per cent for staff with effective CS. Burnout is associated with ineffective CS.

A similar picture emerges from the Minnesota Job Satisfaction data. Staff who rate their CS as ineffective are less likely to have high intrinsic job satisfaction, 5.7 per cent versus 14.7 per cent for effective CS. Total job satisfaction is also lower in ineffective CS, with 8.7 per cent of ineffective staff reporting high job satisfaction, compared with a figure of 14 per cent for staff reporting effective CS.

Both the above studies suggest that the MCSS is the reliable and valid scale that its developers claim. The existence of such a scale enables researchers to conduct more sophisticated studies of CS.

Additional Measures for Evaluating Clinical Supervision

In the previous edition of this book, I recommended five scales that might be suitable for evaluating the process of clinical supervision. These were the Nurse Stress Index, the Maslach Burnout Inventory, the General Health Questionnaire, the Cooper Coping Skills Subscale and the Minnesota Job Satisfaction Scale. These were the measures used in the Clinical Supervision Evaluation Project (Butterworth et al., 1997). Of these five measures, we only found the Maslach Burnout Inventory and the Minnesota Job Satisfaction Scale to be sensitive to change. Interestingly, these were the two measures chosen by Hyrkäs (2005) in the study described above, alongside the MCSS. I will describe both these scales below, as they will be of benefit to other researchers evaluating the process of CS.

The Maslach Burnout Inventory

The concept of burnout is best described by Schaufeli and Enzmann (1998). They state,

> Burnout is a persistent, negative, work-related state of mind in normal individuals, primarily characterised by emotional

exhaustion, which is accompanied by distress, a sense of reduced effectiveness, decreased motivation, and the development of dysfunctional attitudes and behaviours at work. This psychological condition develops gradually but may remain unnoticed by the individual involved. It results from a misfit between intentions and reality in the job. Often burnout is self-perpetuating because of inadequate coping strategies that are often associated with the condition. (p. 36)

While there are a number of scales that have been developed to measure occupational burnout syndrome, the scale that has been most widely utilised is the Maslach Burnout Inventory (Maslach and Jackson, 1986). The scale has twenty-two items that cover the three independent dimensions of the occupational burnout syndrome. These are, Emotional Exhaustion, Depersonalisation and Personal Accomplishment. All items are rated on a seven-point frequency of occurrence scale from 0 = never to 6 = every day. The Emotional Exhaustion subscale has nine items such as, '*I feel emotionally drained from my work*', '*Working with people all day is really a strain for me*', Depersonalisation has five items, for example, '*I can easily understand how my recipients feel about things*', '*I've become more callous towards people since I took this job*', and Personal Accomplishment which has eight items, '*I deal very effectively with the problems of my recipients*', '*I have accomplished many worthwhile things in this job*'. The Maslach Scale has high internal consistency and high test–retest reliability. Its validity has been well established (Sandoval, 1989; Schaufeli and Enzmann, 1998).

Two types of score are obtained from each subscale. First, a total subscale score. Second, a categorical score, which is whether a person has a high, moderate or low burnout score on a particular dimension. A member of staff with a high burnout profile would score high on Emotional Exhaustion, high on Depersonalisation and low on Personal Accomplishment. An analysis of over 600 ward-based mental health nurses showed that only 5 per cent of the total were high on burnout (Fagin et al., 1996). A more recent study of 510 Scottish mental health nurses (Kilfedder et al., 2001), found an even lower percentage to be of high burnout. Large percentages of nurses are found to score highly on Emotional Exhaustion.

While the Maslach Scale does not address the process of CS directly, it helps assess the restorative component of clinical supervision. We might expect that nurses who are well supervised would have lower occupational burnout than nurses without such support. This was indeed one of the findings of the Hyrkäs (2005) study.

Minnesota Job Satisfaction Scale

This scale was developed at the University of Minnesota in the 1960s (Weiss et al., 1967). It was based on Herzberg's theory of work motivation (Herzberg et al., 1959). Herzberg claimed that five factors influenced job satisfaction. These were the intrinsic satisfaction of the job, advancement or professional growth, responsibility, recognition and achievement. Five factors were said to influence job dissatisfaction. These were company policy and administration, supervision, salary, interpersonal relations and working conditions. Job satisfaction factors are all concerned with the job content, while dissatisfaction factors relate to the job environment or context. Weiss and colleagues operationalised these factors into the Minnesota Scale. Three scores are obtained. Intrinsic Satisfaction has twelve items, for example, 'The feeling of accomplishment I get from doing the job', and 'The chance to do things for other people'. Extrinsic satisfaction has six items, for example, 'My pay and the amount of work I do', and 'The competence of my supervisor in making decisions'. Two items do not load on either factor, but are included in calculating the total job satisfaction score. Items are rated on a five-point scale from 1 = very dissatisfied to 5 = very satisfied. The reliability and validity of this scale has been established with nurses in America (Koelbel et al., 1991) and in Britain (Waite et al., 1996). While only one question directly relates to supervision, the scale can be used to evaluate CS as it taps into the normative element of the Proctor model. Again we might hypothesise that staff who receive high quality supervision will have higher levels of job satisfaction. This was also a finding from the Hyrkäs (2005) study.

Clinical Supervision in Special Hospital Nurses

Along with Professor Gournay and other colleagues, I was involved in conducting the Special Hospitals Nursing Staff Stress Survey. This was a questionnaire-based study of nursing staff in Ashworth, Broadmoor and Rampton Hospitals in England and Carstairs in Scotland. While response rates to this survey were low, ranging from 22 to 28 per cent, some 636 nurses participated in the study making it the largest survey of its kind with forensic nurses. The survey used a range of standardised measures of the stress process (Carson and Kuipers, 1998). Stressors were assessed by the Perceived Stress Scale, potential moderators by the Rosenberg Self-Esteem Scale and the PsychNurses Methods of Coping Questionnaire and stress outcomes by the General Health Questionnaire (GHQ-12) and the Minnesota Job Satisfaction Scale. A 52-item background questionnaire was also used. Two of the items on this scale related to CS. These were, 'Are you receiving clinical supervision?' This was answered 'Yes/No'.

Table 7.1 The effects of clinical supervision on stress process measures for special hospital nursing staff

Measures	Clinical Supervision ($n = 282$)	No Supervision ($n = 340$)	t	p value
Stressors				
Present stress Level (0–100)	46.32	48.30	$-.937$	.349
Perceived Stress Scale	17.71	18.78	-2.820	.005
Potential moderators				
Self-confidence (0–100)	73.10	70.13	1.709	.088
Rosenberg Self-esteem	15.39	16.84	-3.832	.000
PsychNurses Coping Scale	125.92	122.43	2.283	.023
Stress outcomes				
GHQ Likert	11.92	13.31	-3.185	.002
Minnesota Extrinsic	16.09	14.66	4.164	.000
Minnesota Intrinsic	39.54	37.33	4.126	.000
Minnesota Total	61.77	57.57	4.798	.000
Sickness absence	11.18	14.69	-1.760	.079

The second asked when staff last received CS. Responses to the first question alone will be considered in the analysis which follows.

Of the sample of nurses surveyed, 50 per cent of the women received CS, in contrast to 43 per cent of the men. Supervision rates varied between the four hospitals ranging from 37 per cent to 54 per cent of staff. Table 7.1 presents the findings on several study variables broken down by whether staff received CS.

Given the large sample size, only findings at the $p<0.01$ level will be reported as significant. This is also a control for multiple statistical comparisons. The above Table 7.1 highlights a number of significant differences between staff who received CS and those who did

Table 7.2 The effects of clinical supervision on stress process measures for male forensic nurses ($n=$ 423)

Measures	Clinical Supervision (n = 181)	No Supervision (n = 242)	t	p value
Stressors				
Present stress Level (0–100)	45.86	48.80	−1.149	.251
Perceived Stress Scale	17.93	18.85	−2.003	.046
Potential moderators				
Self-confidence (0–100)	75.06	72.37	1.293	.197
Rosenberg Self-esteem	15.18	16.62	−3.109	.002
PsychNurses Coping Scale	124.17	120.81	1.751	.081
Stress outcomes				
GHQ Likert	11.58	13.48	−3.587	.000
Minnesota Extrinsic	15.46	14.28	2.908	.004
Minnesota Intrinsic	38.68	37.16	2.246	.025
Minnesota Total	60.31	57.11	2.949	.003
Sickness absence	8.24	13.37	−2.439	.015

Table 7.3 The effects of clinical supervision on stress process measures for female forensic nurses ($n = 195$)

Measures	Clinical Supervision ($n = 98$)	No Supervision ($n = 97$)	t	p value
Stressors				
Present Stress Level (0–100)	46.93	47.03	−.025	.980
Perceived Stress Scale	17.26	18.57	−1.885	.061
Potential moderators				
Self-confidence (0–100)	69.65	64.34	1.673	.096
Rosenberg Self-esteem	15.66	17.25	−2.381	.018
PsychNurses Coping Scale	128.68	126.41	.919	.359
Stress outcomes				
GHQ Likert	12.62	12.92	−.363	.717
Minnesota Extrinsic	17.18	15.58	2.564	.011
Minnesota Intrinsic	41.04	37.74	3.950	.000
Minnesota Total	64.33	58.87	3.719	.000
Sickness Absence	16.92	18.14	−.274	.785

not. Staff who received CS had significantly lower Perceived Stress scores and lower GHQ Likert scores. They also had better levels of self-esteem and higher job satisfaction scores. Apart from asking what benefits accrue to staff from CS, it is also possible to explore sex differences in the response to CS. In brief, do men show a better response to CS than women?

Tables 7.2 and 7.3, both show that male and female forensic nurses who received CS, benefited more than their colleagues who never received CS. While proportionately more women received CS, men did in fact obtain greater clinical benefit from CS than women. Men scored significantly higher on self-esteem, lower on psychological distress and had higher extrinsic and total job satisfaction. Women who received CS scored significantly higher on intrinsic and total job satisfaction.

The Special Hospitals' Nursing Staff Stress Survey has revealed significantly lower levels of job satisfaction among forensic nurses when compared to other groups of inpatient nurses (Carson, 2005). The brief data analysis described above shows that staff in receipt of CS had higher levels of job satisfaction than nurses receiving no CS. Providing more CS to Special Hospital nurses might be one way of increasing their levels of job satisfaction.

Conclusion

There has been considerable progress in evaluating clinical supervision since the first edition of this book was published. The most important development has been the publication of the Manchester Clinical Supervision Scale. This enables an accurate assessment of the quality of clinical supervision provided to staff. This scale has already been used in independent research. Good clinical supervision needs to cover Proctor's three elements of normative, formative and restorative. The Manchester Scale covers all three elements for the first time in one scale. Researchers wanting to evaluate the process of supervision will also find the Maslach Burnout Inventory and the Minnesota Job Satisfaction Scale a useful complement to the Manchester Scale. As a clinical psychologist it is interesting to note that nursing research in clinical supervision is considerably more advanced than clinical supervision research in clinical psychology and psychiatry (Scaife, 2001; MacDonald, 2002; Milne and James, 2005). Perhaps more sad, is the fact that psychologists and psychiatrists are unaware of studies such as the Clinical Supervision Evaluation Project or the existence of the Manchester Clinical Supervision Scale.

Appendix

The Manchester Clinical Supervision Scale can be obtained from the website, clinicalsupervisionscale.com

The Maslach Burnout Inventory can be obtained from Oxford Psychologists, Lambourne House, 311–321 Banbury Road, Oxford OX2 7JH. Tel (01865–510203).

The Minnesota Job Satisfaction Scale is now out of print. Readers interested in obtaining a copy should write to me at the Psychology Department, Henry Wellcome Building, Institute of Psychiatry, De Crespigny Park, Denmark Hill, London SE5 8AF or e-mail me on Jerome.Carson@slam.nhs.uk or JeromeCar@aol.com

References

Brown D, Leary J, Carson J, Bartlett H and Fagin L (1995) Stress and the community metal health nurse: the development of a measure. *Journal of Psychiatric and Mental Health Nursing*, 2(1): 9–12.

Burnard P, Edwards D, Hannigan B, Fothergill A and Coyle D (2000) Report of the findings of the all-Wales survey of stress among community mental health nurses. Cardiff: School of Nursing, Midwifery and Health Visiting, University of Wales.

Butterworth T (1996) Primary attempts at research based evaluation of clinical supervision. *NT Research*, 1(2): 96–101.

Butterworth T and Faugier J (1992) Supervision for life. In: Butterworth T and Faugier J (eds), *Clinical Supervision and Mentorship in Nursing*. Chapman and Hall, London.

Butterworth T, Carson J, White E, Jeacock J, Clements A and Bishop V (1997) It is good to talk: An evaluation study in England and Scotland. Manchester: School of Nursing, Midwifery and Health Visiting, University of Manchester.

Carson J (2005) The Stress Process in Mental Health Workers: Assessment and Intervention Studies. Unpublished doctoral thesis, King's College, University of London.

Carson J and Kuipers E (1998) Stress management interventions. In: Hardy S, Carson J and Thomas B (eds) *Occupational Stress: Personal and Professional Approaches*. Stanley Thornes, Cheltenham.

Cooper C, Sloan S and Williams S (1988) *The Occupational Stress Indicator*. NFER-Nelson, Windsor.

Cronbach L (1951) Co-efficient alpha and the internal consistency of tests. *Psychometrika*, 16: 297–334.

Department of Health (2000) *Making a Difference: Clinical Supervision in Primary Care*. HMSO, London.

Edwards D, Cooper L, Burnard P, Hannigan B, Adams J, Fothergill A and Coyle D (2005) Factors influencing the effectiveness of clinical supervision. *Journal of Psychiatric and Mental Health Nursing*, 12: 405–414.

Eysenck H (1980) The bio-social model of man and the unification of psychology. In: Chapman A and Jones D (eds), *Models of Man*. British Psychological Society, Leicester.

Eysenck H and Eysenck S (1975) Manual for the Eysenck Personality Questionnaire. Hodder and Stoughton, London.

Fagin L, Carson J, Leary J, De Villiers N, Bartlett H, O'Malley P, West M, McElfatrick S and Brown D (1996) Stress, coping and burnout in mental health nurses: findings from three research studies. *The International Journal of Social Psychiatry*, 42(2): 102–111.

Faugier J (1996) Clinical supervision and mental health nursing. In: Sandford T and Gournay K (eds) *Perspectives in Mental Health Nursing*. Balliere Tindall, London.

Foster J (1998) Data Analysis Using SPSS for Windows. Sage, London.

Goldberg D and Williams S (1988) A User's Guide to the General Health Questionnaire. NFER-Nelson, Windsor.

Goering P and Streiner D (1996) Reconcilable differences: the marriage of qualitative and quantitative methods. *Canadian Journal of Psychiatry*, 41(8): 491–497.

Green D (1995) Supervision for qualified clinical psychologists. *Clinical Psychology Forum*, 80: 40–41.

Harris P (1989) The Nurse Stress Index. *Work and Stress*, 5(4): 335–346.

Herzberg F, Mausner B and Snyderman B (1959) *The Motivation to Work*. Chapman and Hall, London.

Holloway E (1995) *Clinical Supervision: A Systems Approach*. Sage, California.

Hyrkäs K (2005) Clinical supervision, burnout and job satisfaction among mental health and psychiatric nurses in Finland. *Issues in Mental Health Nursing*, 26: 531–556.

Kilfedder C, Power K and Wells T (2001) Burnout in psychiatric nursing. *Journal of Advanced Nursing*, 34(3): 383–396.

Kinnear P and Gray C (1994) *SPSS for Windows Made Simple*. Lawrence Erlbaum, Hove.

Koelbel P, Fuller F and Misener T (1991) Job satisfaction of nurse practitioners: an analysis using Herzberg's theory. *Nurse Practitioner*, 16(4): 43–46.

MacDonald J (2002) Clinical supervision: a review of underlying concepts and developments. *Australian and New Zealand Journal of Psychiatry*, 36: 92–98.

Mann S and Cowburn J (2005) Emotional labour and stress within mental health nursing. *Journal of Psychiatric and Mental Health Nursing*, 12: 154–162.

Maslach C and Jackson S (1986) *Maslach Burnout Inventory*. Consulting Psychologists Press, California.

Milne D and James I (2005) Clinical supervision: ten tests of the tandem model. *Clinical Psychology Forum*, 151: 6–9.

Norussis M (1993) SPSS for Windows: Base System User's Guide. SPSS Inc., Chicago.

Proctor B (1986) Supervision: a co-operative exercise in accountability. In: Marken A and Payne M (eds), *Enabling and Ensuring: Supervision in Practice*. National Youth Bureau, Leicester.

Proctor B and Inskipp F (2001) Group supervision. In: Scaife J (ed), *Supervision in the Mental Health Professions: A Practitioner's Guide*. Brunner Routledge, Hove.

Ritter S, Norman I, Rentoul L and Bodley D (1996) A model of clinical supervision for nurses undertaking short placements in mental health care settings. *Journal of Clinical Nursing*, 5: 149–158.

Rust J and Golombok S (1989) *Modern Psychometrics: The Science of Psychological Assessment*. Routledge, London.

Sandoval J (1989) Review of the Maslach Burnout Inventory. In: Close-Caroly K and Kramer J (eds), *Mental Measurement Yearbook 10*. Buros Institute of Mental Measurement, Lincoln, Nebraska.

Scaife J (2001) (Ed) *Supervision in the Mental Health Professions: A Practitioner's Guide*. Brunner Routledge, Hove.

Schaufeli W and Enzmann D (1998) *The Burnout Companion to Study and Practice: A Critical Analysis*. Taylor and Francis, London.

Simms J (1993) Supervision. In: Wright H and Giddey M (eds), *Mental Health Nursing: From First Principles to Professional Practice*. Chapman and Hall, London.

Streiner D (1990) Sample size and power in psychiatric research. *Canadian Journal of Psychiatry*, 35(7): 616–620.

Streiner D (1993a) A checklist for evaluating the usefulness of rating scales. *Canadian Journal of Psychiatry*, 38(2): 140–148.

Streiner D (1993b) An introduction to multivariate statistics. *Canadian Journal of Psychiatry*, 38(2): 9–13.

Streiner D (1994) Figuring out factors: the use and misuse of factor analysis. *Canadian Journal of Psychiatry*, 39(3): 135–140.

Streiner D (1995) Learning how to differ: agreement and reliability statistics in psychiatry. *Canadian Journal of Psychiatry*, 40(2): 60–66.

Streiner D (1996a) While you're up get me a grant: a guide to grant writing. *Canadian Journal of Psychiatry*, 41(3): 137–143.

Streiner D (1996b) Maintaining standards: differences between the standard deviation and standard error and when to use each. *Canadian Journal of Psychiatry*, 41(8): 489–501.

Streiner D (2000a) The case of the missing data: methods of dealing with dropouts and other research vagaries. *Canadian Journal of Psychiatry*, 47: 68–75.

Streiner D (2000b) Breaking up is hard to do: the heartbreak of dichotomising continuous data. *Canadian Journal of Psychiatry*, 47(3): 262–265.

Streiner D (2002c) The 2 E's of research: efficacy and effectiveness trials. *Canadian Journal of Psychiatry*, 47(6): 552–556.

Streiner D and Norman G (1989) *Health Measurement Scales: A Practical Guide to Their Development and Use*. Oxford University Press, Oxford.

UKCC (United Kingdom Central Council for Nursing, Midwifery and Health Visiting) (1996) Position Statement on Clinical Supervision for Nursing, Midwifery and Health Visiting. UKCC, London.

Waite A, Oliver N, Carson J and Fagin L (1996) Mental health nursing: is community or ward based nursing more satisfying? *Psychiatric Care*, 2(5): 167–170.

Weiss D, Dawis R, England G and Lofquist L (1967) Manual for the Minnesota Satisfaction Questionnaire. Industrial Relations Centre, University of Minnesota.

White E, Butterworth T, Bishop V, Carson J, Jeacock J and Clements A (1998) Clinical supervision: insider reports of a private world. *Journal of Advanced Nursing*, 8(1): 85–102.

Winstanley J (2000) Manchester Clinical Supervision Scale. *Nursing Standard*, 14(19): 31–32.

Winstanley J and White E (2003) Clinical supervision: models, measures and best practice. *Nurse Researcher*, 10(4): 7–38.

Index